T0261429

Interprofessional Education and Collaboration

An Evidence-Based Approach to Optimizing Health Care

Jordan Hamson-Utley PhD, LAT, ATC
University of St. Augustine

Cynthia Kay Mathena, PhD, OTR/L
University of St. Augustine

Tina Patel Gunaldo, PhD, DPT, MHS
Louisiana State University Health–New Orleans

EDITORS

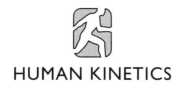

HUMAN KINETICS

Library of Congress Cataloging-in-Publication Data

Names: Hamson-Utley, Jennifer Jordan, editor. | Mathena, Cynthia Kay, 1963-
editor. | Gunaldo, Tina Patel, 1972- editor.
Title: Interprofessional education and collaboration : an evidence-based
approach to optimizing health care / [edited by] J. Jordan Hamson-Utley,
Cynthia Kay Mathena, Tina Patel Gunaldo.
Description: First. | Champaign, IL : Human Kinetics, Inc., [2021] |
Includes bibliographical references and index.
Identifiers: LCCN 2019038044 (print) | LCCN 2019038045 (ebook) | ISBN
9781492590033 (print) | ISBN 9781492593188 (epub) | ISBN 9781492593171
(pdf)
Subjects: MESH: Interprofessional Relations | Interdisciplinary Placement
Classification: LCC RA425 (print) | LCC RA425 (ebook) | NLM W 62 | DDC
362.1--dc23
LC record available at https://lccn.loc.gov/2019038044
LC ebook record available at https://lccn.loc.gov/2019038045

ISBN: 978-1-4925-9003-3 (print)

Acquisitions Editor: Joshua J. Stone; **Developmental and Managing Editor:** Amanda S. Ewing; **Copyeditor:** Alisha Jeddeloh; **Indexer:** Rebecca L. McCorkle; **Permissions Manager:** Dalene Reeder; **Graphic Designer:** Julie L. Denzer; **Cover Designer:** Keri Evans; **Cover Design Specialist:** Susan Rothermel Allen; **Photographs (cover):** Jeffrey Collingwood/ fotolia.com and © Human Kinetics; **Photo Production Manager:** Jason Allen; **Senior Art Manager:** Kelly Hendren; **Illustrations:** © Human Kinetics, unless otherwise noted; **Printer:** Versa Press

Printed in the United States of America   10 9 8 7 6 5 4 3 2 1

The paper in this book is certified under a sustainable forestry program.

Human Kinetics
1607 N. Market St.
Champaign, IL 61820
Website: www.HumanKinetics.com

In the United States, email info@hkusa.com or call 800-747-4457.
In Canada, email info@hkcanada.com.
In the United Kingdom/Europe, email hk@hkeurope.com.

For information about Human Kinetics' coverage in other areas of the world,
please visit our website: **www.HumanKinetics.com**

E7484

Tell us what you think!
Human Kinetics would love to hear what we
can do to improve the customer experience.
Use this QR code to take our brief survey.

To my family and friends for your constant support of my next endeavor. You provide the gas that fuels the adventure (to the end), the map that keeps me on the high side of the road (and out of the ditch), and the reasons to push harder for change. To Michael and Seth, thank you for supporting me through the completion of another book. Only you know the sacrifices. Love you!

—Jordan

The work that went into this book was the result of collegial and collaborative support from respected colleagues. I have much gratitude for each of you. Thank you to my parents who provided the foundation and backdrop to my passion for inquiry. I dedicate this book to my son, Dillon, who inspires me in every effort I make to be bold in making change.

—Cindy

To Mike, Misha, Jbhai, and Maya. None of my accomplishments would have been realized without your support and understanding. To Sandra and Al, thank you for including me in your journey.

—Tina

The editors would like to recognize Josh Stone for his early vision on this project as an essential and impactful piece for the health care workforce.

Contents

Chapter 7 ▪ **Interprofessional Communication Strategies** . 145

Dee M. Lance, PhD, CCC-SLP/L
Kim C. McCullough, PhD, CCC-SLP/L

Chapter 8 ▪ **Building Sustainability**. .163

Tina Patel Gunaldo, PhD, DPT, MHS
Pamela Waynick-Rogers, DNP, APRN-BC

Preface

Today's health care landscape calls for a team approach, which optimizes patient outcomes and quality of care. Health professionals must possess a strong collaborative skill set to function on today's health care teams and meet the goals set by the World Health Organization (WHO). In addition, many program accreditors are calling for evidence of interprofessional competency, demonstrating the importance of and demand for the topic. Thus, *Interprofessional Education in Health Care* is written for educators (in academia or clinical practice), health professionals, and health administrators who are interested in learning more about an interprofessional approach to improving patient and community outcomes. It provides a foundational base for interprofessional education (IPE) and interprofessional collaborative practice (IPCP), including realistic examples applying newly learned knowledge. Each chapter is filled with evidence-based information substantiated by numerous references from various resources and multiple professions. Health professionals who are interested in developing lifelong learning in IPCP will find this textbook to be a detailed yet succinct introduction to IPE and a starting point from which to develop IPCP skills.

IPE literature is growing rapidly, with a call to strengthen the connection between IPE and IPCP. This textbook is a first of its kind in summarizing foundational reports and research in IPE while providing evidence-based practice strategies in IPCP. WHO notes that IPE is a precursor to IPCP. Of specific interest, this book focuses on developing intentional behaviors that will assist in gathering evidence, planning, and implementing interprofessional activities designed to improve patient outcomes. These skills, along with conflict resolution and other essential ingredients, promote collaboration in the workplace. Current educators in the health science fields are in a unique position to shape the future of health care through an interprofessional curriculum, exposing students to real-life collaborative care teams through innovative educational experiences (e.g., simulation). The textbook summarizes evidence-based pedagogies to date and offers strategies for implementation.

Beginning with basic definitions, this textbook serves as a foundational guide to IPE and IPCP, meeting the needs of educators across professions. Essential topics such as creating a culture for teams, building interprofessional relationships, and fostering collaboration build to topics such as leading interprofessional teams, managing conflict, and sustaining the interprofessional effort. Case studies and collaborative activities round out the textbook, creating a true handbook feeling.

Organization

The textbook is organized by chapter themes, one chapter building on the next to expand the reader's knowledge and interprofessional skills. With intention, each chapter stands on its own, creating a modular approach to professional development of existing teams in the workplace.

This textbook provides a foundation for IPE and IPCP. The evidence-based information provided in each chapter is substantiated by numerous references from various resources and multiple professions. The content can be utilized in whole or in part based on the needs of the reader, and the language surrounding interprofessional teams is intentionally neutral and inclusive.

The chapters of the book are intentionally divided to provide information on IPE and IPCP separately, based on the current research. Chapters 1 through 4 cover evidence related to IPE, and chapters 5 through 8 focus more on IPCP.

- Chapter 1 provides a strong foundation for IPE and IPCP by examining the historical underpinnings and mapping decades of collaborative actions across health professions. This chapter also provides essential definitions for the study of IPE and IPCP.
- Chapter 2 advances the reader into models of IPE delivery by highlighting how the pre- and postlicense clinician develops a collaborative skill set and a dual identity (both professional and team-based).
- Chapter 3 expands beyond the student learner to developing the same skills in clinician preceptors (clinical instructors and field work supervisors) and faculty. The environment and IPE facilitator skills are a special focus of this chapter.
- Chapter 4 takes a deep dive into the evidence surrounding IPE and IPCP as it relates to the global goals of the Triple Aim. The chapter also presents Kirkpatrick's Typology as applied to IPE and IPCP and provides a summary of various tools to assess IPE and IPCP.
- While Chapter 5 highlights elements of interprofessional relationship building within teams that already exist (and new teams), chapter 6 gets at the science of teaming and how IPCP can drive change in behaviors associated with care delivery. Communication is essential, whether it be within or across professions.
- Chapter 7 links effective communication with team-based care strategies to reach the goals set in chapter 1 by the Triple Aim.
- Chapter 8 rounds out the textbook with a focus on sustaining both IPE and IPCP efforts. This chapter examines goals, resources, and strategy related to IPE and IPCP initiatives and offers guidance through industry-relevant frameworks.

As a health professional, it is important to understand what research has been conducted in both academic and clinical environments, because education will influence practice, and practice should influence the delivery of education. The health industry has much more to learn about IPE and IPCP, but as champions in this area, we are all dedicated to discovering and employing evidence-based practices to improve the health of the communities we serve.

Unique Features

This textbook offers unique learning opportunities. Most important is the professional diversity of the authors, who represent 7 professions: athletic training, dietetics, industrial engineering, nursing, occupational therapy (OT), physical therapy (PT), and speech language pathology (SLP). Throughout the book, the reader will be exposed to multiple resources, such as major IPE and IPCP stakeholders. Take time to visit the websites of the various organizations; they are a source of additional information and offer opportunities to engage with others interested in this emerging area.

To help readers take theoretical concepts and apply them in the real world, we have created some unique features.

- *EBP of Teamship*—This feature will guide the reader by showcasing current findings (in abbreviated abstract form) on IPE and ICPC related to the chapter topics.

- *Tools of IPE*—This feature highlights specific IPE and IPCP tools related to the chapter topics. Tools include surveys, inventories, and activities that educators, students, and health care providers might implement in their daily practice.

- *Collaborative Corner*—This feature provides reflective questions or statements regarding IPE and IPCP as related to the chapter content. Readers should take advantage of the interprofessional learning that can occur when various perspectives are shared among the team while working through the Collaborative Corner features together.

- *Case Studies*—Each chapter begins with a case study incorporating IPE or IPCP. At the closing of the chapter is a debriefing that explains the case studies and poses discussion questions.

These unique additions support practical application of the chapter content. Readers should revisit these areas over time to reflect on new perspectives as they grow interprofessionally. Student or clinical teams should also take advantage of the learning that can occur when using the case studies, Collaborative Corner, and Evidence-Based Practice sidebars as IPE activities.

Instructor Ancillaries

Two ancillaries are provided for instructors.

- *Instructor guide*—The instructor guide contains a sample course outline and syllabus; Signature Assessments, which are designed to assess mastery of the chapter content; a list of additional resources; and chapter-specific files that contain a chapter summary, team activities, and discussion questions.

- *Image bank*—The image bank provides most figures and tables from the text, sorted by chapter. Instructors can use the image bank to enhance lectures, create handouts, build slideshow presentations, and more.

The instructor ancillaries are available at www.HumanKinetics.com/InterprofessionalEducationAndCollaboration.

CHAPTER 1

Interprofessional Health Care

Cindy Mathena, PhD, OTR/L

Objectives

After reading this chapter, the reader will be able to do the following:

- Define key concepts and terms related to interprofessional health care delivery.
- Articulate the importance of a collaborative approach to health care delivery.
- Discuss enabling factors for and barriers to implementation of collaborative practice.
- Trace the history of interprofessional education and collaborative practice.
- Describe key organizations and resources supporting interprofessional health care approaches.

CASE STUDY Getting Teams to Talk

Russell is a 46-year-old male with a diagnosis of amyotrophic lateral sclerosis (ALS). Since his diagnosis approximately a year ago, Russell has experienced an overall decline in muscle function, with recent difficulty in chewing and swallowing. He has also rapidly lost the quality and volume of his speech production, and he now requires full assistance with all activities of daily living (ADLs). In a recent discussion with Russell's physician, the family has decided to use a power wheelchair as the primary method of mobility and to use voice recognition software and adaptive switches for accessing the computer. Additionally, there have been discussions about using a feeding tube for nutritional intake because Russell is losing weight. He has now entered a rehabilitation facility to receive a comprehensive suite of evaluations and interventions to optimize his independence at home.

(continued)

Case Study *(continued)*

Russell is married with two teenage daughters. Three months ago, he decided to leave his job as an information technology executive for a large advertising firm. He felt he was no longer valuable to the company and required too much assistance from others while at work. His wife states she is performing the majority of Russell's ADLs, and she recently began feeding him milkshakes because eating seems to "take a lot of energy and is messy, and he coughs a lot." This latter information is not shared with anyone other than the psychologist, who is working with the family on coping strategies.

Upon entering the rehabilitation facility, Russell is evaluated by professionals from numerous fields, including a nurse, occupational therapist (OT), physical therapist (PT), speech language pathologist (SLP), social worker, and nutritionist. Each professional completes the initial evaluations and documents findings in the electronic medical record (EMR) system. These evaluations are readily accessible to all providers involved in Russell's care. A nurse documents "difficulty eating with increased coughing and choking during meals," while the SLP professional observes that "signs of aspiration are present during vocalizations." The physical therapist notes Russell is "experiencing difficulty with the stamina necessary for feeding himself," while the occupational therapist documents the need for "adaptive devices to assist with positioning and self-feeding."

On Friday after a week of therapy, the SLP staff member indicates Russell is displaying signs of aspiration and labored breathing. She observes him eating and is concerned he is aspirating some of his food while attempting to swallow. She calls the physician, informs the nurse of the possible aspiration, and leaves instructions for a feeding protocol in the EMR. The occupational therapist also documents concerns and recommends additional measures for ensuring safe positioning for feeding. Over the weekend, nurses report that Russell enjoyed time with his family and fully participated in therapy. He ate several meals both with family and with a certified nursing assistant (CNA). On Sunday evening, a nurse reports that Russell is febrile, his breathing is labored, and he is generally unresponsive. Diagnostics reveal he has severe pneumonia, and he is immediately transferred to the intensive care unit (ICU), where he later passes away.

As tragic as this case might be, it speaks to the basic need for communication and teamwork. Professionals cannot expect siloed, episodic treatments to be an effective way to care for the complex needs of a patient. In the end, Russell's health could have been managed by any number of interventions, including a feeding tube, proper feeding adaptations (pureed food), and proper feeding techniques. During a debriefing of the situation, it was determined that the professionals only read the reports of their specific discipline and did not read the reports of the other health care disciplines. Within each professional silo, the health care worker was probably acting with appropriate expertise and interventions; however, lack of communication over the course of the weekend led to this tragic scenario. If the professionals had collaborated on a plan of care and interventions, the outcome might have been very different. Interviews and quality assurance reviews revealed that the professionals involved in Russell's care missed opportunities to plan for and deliver a holistic, collaborative approach to safe health care.

COLLABORATIVE CORNER
Speaking the Same Professional Language

What were the missed opportunities for Russell's treatment in the opening case example? Let's first determine if everyone was using the same language. For example, *fatigue, positioning, choking*, and *coughing* are all terms used in the case example that describe contributors to aspiration. These are common words, not necessarily used by any one profession. Although the health professionals documented the potential cause of aspiration related to treatment intervention in their specific disciplines, they never addressed preventing aspiration as a team. Using common language to describe findings supports a collaborative approach. Speaking the same language or understanding that of the other professions might be the basis for a collaborative approach. One way to overcome siloed documentation and treatment is to incorporate team discussions when a major concern, such as aspiration, is identified by a provider. The team could agree upon terminologies to use in communications, including with the patient and family. What other methods or activities might assist in understanding a common language?

Cases such as the one described here will be the cornerstone of this textbook, allowing the reader to begin translating the impact of interprofessional education (IPE) on interprofessional collaborative practice (IPCP). These cases will help educators and health professionals take a thoughtful approach to gathering evidence, planning and implementing interprofessional activities, and ultimately improving patient outcomes. Educators are in a unique position to shape the future of health care through an interprofessional approach to curriculum design, exposing learners to collaborative teams through innovative educational experiences (e.g., simulation) and by championing IPE and IPCP as transformative causes. This chapter will outline the foundational concepts of IPCP and IPE, explain common terminologies, and establish the importance of collaborative care.

Communication and Teamwork

As can be seen in the case of Russell, effective IPCP, specifically communication and teamwork, may be the most critical aspect of successful health care. Exchange of information during every step of the health care process is crucial to achieving collaborative care, and the lack of exchange can be important, if not critical, to proper care.[1]

> Interprofessional Communication is especially important, as the exchange of information is a critical factor in all phases of collaborative patient care, and the impact of this exchange—or lack of exchange—can be profound.[1(p3)]

Studies indicate that ineffectual communication among health care providers may be a direct contributor to patient injury. Some organizations have called for change in the U.S. health care system, due to poor communication and teamwork leading to medical errors. One such organization, formerly the Institute of Medicine, now known as the National Academy of Medicine (NAM), has produced multiple reports outlining methods for improving health care quality. In 2003, NAM introduced the idea that teamwork would improve patient care, noting that when professionals have appropriate communication and comprehend each worker's unique role, they work more effectively as a team.[2]

The Joint Commission on Accreditation of Healthcare Organizations, an organization focused on improving quality care, recognized the criticality of effective and efficient communication between health care professionals. Their research indicates that more than 70% of sentinel medical errors may be traced to communication failures.[3] What's more, teams sharing a common language and embracing a common communication process have been attributed to safer and more efficient care.[4]

A prevalent example of discipline-specific terminology is descriptors related to patient transfers. A PT may describe the transfer as a "pivot transfer from seated on bed to wheelchair performed with moderate assist." Nursing staff may describe the transfer as "bed to chair with hand-hold assist." These phrases may or may not equate to the same objective findings, but nevertheless they are subjective and may mean something different to each discipline. If they are not understood, the transfer may not be performed with the appropriate amount of assistance by another professional, putting the patient at risk for a fall or accident.

Uniform Terminology

A review of common terminology will be helpful to further frame the conversation. In its Framework for Action on Interprofessional Education and Collaborative Practice (figure 1.1), the World Health Organization (WHO)[5] outlines key terminology for consideration:

- **collaborative practice-ready health workforce**—One in which "staff work together to provide comprehensive services in a wide range of health-care settings."[5(p13)]

- **health and education systems**—"Organizations, people and actions whose primary intent is to promote, restore or maintain health and facilitate learning, respectively."[5(p13)]

- **health worker**—"A person whose primary intent is to enhance health,"[5(p13)] or one who promotes and preserves health, diagnoses and treats disease, performs health management, and supports workers, as well as others who contribute to the overall health or wellness of a person or group of people. For this book, health workers are further defined as the professionals who provide direct health care (whether primary or rehabilitative) and may include physicians, nurses, OTs, speech therapists, PTs, athletic trainers, nutritionists, social workers, and PAs.

- **interprofessional collaborative practice (IPCP)**—"Multiple health workers from different professional backgrounds working together with patients, families, caregivers, and communities to deliver the highest quality of care."[5(p13)]

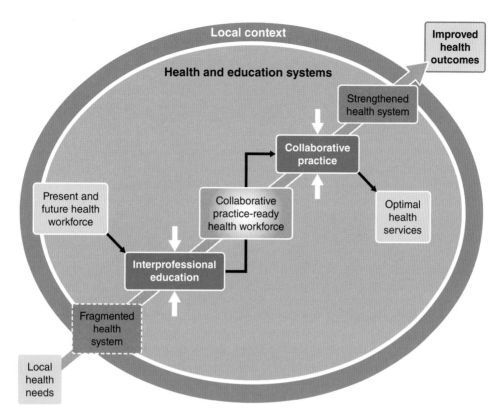

Figure 1.1   Framework for Action on Interprofessional Education and Collaborative Practice. The diagram shows how IPE is essential in preparing practice-ready health care workers who will use collaborative practice to provide a more optimal delivery model in solving health needs and improving health outcomes.

Reprinted from *Framework for Action on Interprofessional Education & Collaborative Practice*, World Health Organization, pg. 18., Copyright 2010.

- **interprofessional education (IPE)**—"Occurs when two or more professions learn about, from and with each other to enable effective collaboration and improve health outcomes."[5(p13)] The goal of IPE is, according to WHO, a "collaborative practice-ready health workforce."

- **multiprofessional education (MPE)**—The process by which a group of students (or workers) in health-related fields and with different educational backgrounds learn together during certain periods of their education. MPE is generally thought of as a precursor to IPE and IPCP.[25]

Importance of Collaboration

The fictional case of Russell highlights the need for a collaborative health care workforce and, maybe even more importantly, the need for distinct competencies—such as communication, teamwork, and collaboration—to be adopted and

> ### EBP OF TEAMSHIP
> ### IPE and IPCP as Necessary Components of Patient Safety and Effective Communication
>
> A systematic review of the literature evaluated the effectiveness of IPE and provided the following relevant conclusions: IPE implementation increased student understanding and performance on interprofessional collaboration, and implementation of IPE in practice improved patient satisfaction and health care outcomes.[4] IPCP is necessary to address patient safety and to deal with a complex health care system, including current resources with both human and financial shortages.

integrated so health care practitioners will be ready for practice. A collaborative practice-ready workforce arguably might be positioned to avoid, if not eliminate, poor patient outcomes such as Russell's. Health care professionals, educators, and administrators are increasingly interested in understanding how IPCP may contribute to better patient outcomes. No single provider can deliver the care needed for today's complex health care needs, and IPCP and IPE have been documented as a means for solving health care issues.[4,6] A growing body of literature exists to support the need for transformative education and practice.

Enablers and Barriers of IPCP and IPE

WHO, along with other sources, has identified enablers of and barriers to effective IPCP and IPE (figure 1.2) in its Framework for Action on Interprofessional Education and Collaborative Practice.[5] These items align with those identified in other studies, such as recognition of perceived barriers and enablers in IPE for medical and nursing students.[7] A qualitative study attempted to identify the specific factors, both positive and negative, that influenced IPE effectiveness.

- Enablers included the promotion of interprofessional thinking and acting, promotion of mutual understanding, and reduction of hierarchies.
- Barriers included standardization of learning content levels, differing levels of knowledge, lack of or low respect between medical and nursing students, and capacity and legal issues.

Overall the number of enablers was higher than the number of barriers.[7]

Enablers

Several literature sources discuss enablers of IPE and IPCP. These include leadership, maximization of resources to solve complex problems, institutional support, shared vision, mentoring and learning, and an "enabling built environment."[7(p2)] To remain feasible under new models of reimbursement, such as value-based care, health care

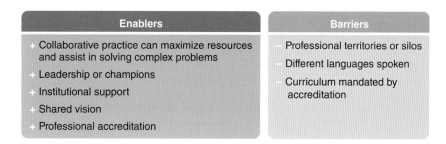

Enablers	Barriers
+ Collaborative practice can maximize resources and assist in solving complex problems	− Professional territories or silos
+ Leadership or champions	− Different languages spoken
+ Institutional support	− Curriculum mandated by accreditation
+ Shared vision	
+ Professional accreditation	

Figure 1.2 Enablers and barriers to effective IPCP and IPE as described by the World Health Organization.

professionals must collaborate on patient care and, when feasible, partner with other professions to create a comprehensive approach to health care delivery.[5] The shift from traditional medical care to IPCP presents several benefits or enablers of professional collaboration. When health care professionals are encouraged to come together to solve common problems, or when funding is limited, a collaborative solution presents an opportunity to share resources, and opportunities for collaborative practice are likely to emerge.

> IPE and IPCP maximize the strengths and skills of health workers, enabling them to function at the highest capacity. With a current shortage of 4.3 million health workers, innovations of this nature will become more and more necessary to manage the strain placed on health systems.[5(p15)]

As with any initiative, leaders are important to the cause. A variety of studies note that in university programs with IPE initiatives, faculty champions and leaders who are passionate about collaboration are important enablers in the success of the initiative.[8,9] The success of a program requires leaders and champions to lead the change. In the university setting, this would include faculty, administrators, and students. Student leaders in particular may have a greater influence on their peers in comparison to faculty.[8] Facilitating student leadership appears to be critical to the sustainability of IPE and IPCP and should be an area of focus for institutional leaders.

Strong leaders, whether clinicians, students, faculty, or administrators, will be instrumental in eliciting institutional support. This support may come in a variety of forms, including policy creation, culture facilitation, and resource provision. Institutional support is also necessary for development of a supportive physical environment both in clinical practice and education. Collaborative spaces accommodate a new way of thinking, one that facilitates communication and breaks down barriers. Often in education, this means an area where simulation can occur. Chapters 2 and 3 explore simulation as a physical environment that is ideal for IPE.

If IPE and IPCP will survive and thrive in an environment where leaders are supportive, then perhaps the most important enabler is a shared mission and vision. A shared vision and mission may also be critical to successful collaboration and will set the stage for the planning and implementation that allow IPCP and IPE to be a truly transformational movement. The WHO framework states that a shared vision is essential in the development of curriculum and educational programs.[5]

Many of the cases presented in this textbook will highlight the importance of a shared mission and vision for a team to successfully collaborate. A review of the literature highlights the importance of the shared vision in all stages of development and implementation.[5,7,10-12]

Professional accreditation is uniquely positioned as both an enabler and a barrier:

> Accreditors occupy a unique position, working within and across professions and health care delivery settings to promote interprofessional collaboration in education and care.[15(p2)]

A proposed model of health care accreditation suggests accreditors could work together to facilitate shared values and competencies in an effort to enhance collaboration and achieve the Quadruple Aim.[15,19] The Quadruple Aim builds on the Triple Aim, which is a framework for optimizing health care through improving population health, enhancing the patient care experience, and reducing cost. The fourth aim focuses on the institution-specific priorities typically highlighting provider work life. IPE and IPCP provide a unique opportunity to enable the Quadruple Aim. Shared professional values and competencies promote all 4 of the aims, just as collaboration among accreditors would benefit a common goal of achieving the Quadruple Aim.[15]

Barriers

Just as enablers or opportunities have been outlined in the literature as being necessary for success, some barriers exist as well. Many are obvious and include professional cultures promoting silos or stereotypes, use of different language and terminology, accreditors, and a required prescribed curriculum.[5,7] Students are educated as they always have been, in schools of nursing, colleges of social work, and departments of athletic training. One can walk into any hospital or medical facility and find that tribalism is still alive and well.[13] Nurses are still holding nursing meetings, OTs still have their own department, and PTs are still working at their desks next to each other. This solo work commonly leads one to think of working in a silo. Socialization, communication, IPE, and IPCP are some of the more obvious solutions to this barrier.[9,14]

Collaboration by the health care team can come at a cost and is difficult to achieve in a hierarchical team where some are seen as the leaders (physicians) and others as the team. A large number of studies validate the presence of professional stereotypes and cultures in the health care workplace.[9,13,14] Many argue the solution to silos rests on the shoulders of the educational institution. Learning environments must be created that encourage real-life scenarios where students can learn the complexities of communication and problem solving with other professionals and as a team.

Accreditation requirements can be another barrier, though it should be pointed out that accreditors are also in a position to enable IPE. In the same way we see health care professionals working in a silo, accrediting agencies that certify educational institutions and programs have also historically worked alone. Standards for accreditation are often so prescriptive that little room is left in the curriculum to explore the roles and language of other professionals. Several studies cite limitations in curricula focused on discipline-specific skills and knowledge as a barrier to IPE. Because curricula are often well defined by professional accreditors, integrating other professions and competencies can be challenging.[10,15] If universities and institutions play a primary role in the integration of IPCP into the preparation of students in health care, accreditors may have the biggest opportunity to create impactful IPE. It has been suggested that this would include an intersection of accreditors with overlapping standards.

> Accreditors occupy a unique position, working within and across professions and health care delivery settings to promote interprofessional collaboration in education and care. Those who work within individual health professions and those accreditors working in different health care delivery domains should look to cross professional and delivery divides for more integrated approaches to the evaluation and regulation of education and clinical practice.[15(p2)]

Inconsistent and varying terminologies have been recognized as a barrier to IPCP and IPE. In the authors' experience, we have encountered students across health care professions who claim this to be the most significant barrier to IPCP in the health care setting. And while the terminologies used by each discipline may widely vary, our students state that it is important to begin discussions about these differences in the classroom.

Separate to this conversation about terminology is the need to understand that the interpretation of IPCP and IPE may vary by discipline. One study found that nurses and physicians in the operating room defined *collaboration* very differently. Nurses interpreted it to mean influencing team decisions, whereas physicians interpreted it as meaning their directions would be followed by the other disciplines on the team.[16]

Additional barriers to IPE implementation were noted in a study of nursing and medical students' perceptions of enablers and barriers. Those barriers included varying knowledge levels, low mutual respect between professions, and capacity and legal issues.[7]

COLLABORATIVE CORNER
Importance of Speaking the Same Professional Language

Students often say the most important thing they learn from their IPE courses is how to speak a common language free of discipline-specific terminologies. One student says, "We can all work together to bring the best care to our patients, but we have to learn how to speak with each other, using a language we all understand. I learned in my IPE courses that it takes some effort, but it is well worth it."

Accreditation Approaches

Programmatic or professional accreditors typically prescribe a range of skills and knowledge in standards of accreditation, and schools and programs are challenged to fit everything into a curriculum that is reasonable in length and cost. This, combined with the complex task of scheduling courses and activities in congruence with other programs, may make the challenge seem insurmountable. Certainly, it is more difficult to develop or maintain a curriculum that creates shared experiences for students between disciplines and programs than to offer a homogenous curriculum not requiring one to solve these complexities. The cost of collaboration can be high when you consider the faculty training, specialized facilities, and reallocation of processes and resources that may be required.

Many professional accreditors have now begun to require IPE or the demonstration of collaborative practice competencies. An innovative approach to accreditation has been suggested by a group of accreditors from multiple health professions that met to deliberate the standards for IPE. The accreditors have begun discussing the spectrum of educational standards that should occur in IPE beginning with entry into the professional area of study, spanning graduate education, and extending to continuing professional development.[15]

As mentioned, some programmatic accreditors require educational institutions to demonstrate the use of IPE in their curricula (see chapter 3 for more details). In response, academic programs have developed IPE experiences through case-based studies, simulations, and community projects. However, putting professions side by side in the classroom is only a start, and IPE is much more than simply learning with other health care providers. According to the WHO framework, two categories or mechanisms shape how IPE is delivered:

1. *Educator mechanisms* are those aspects of the delivery that rely on the expertise of the academic faculty and their experiences with IPE, institutional support, and desired learning outcomes. Clinical preceptors are professionals who work with students in the health care environment. They are typically health care providers charged with mentoring students. When preceptors model collaborative practices, they assist in bridging education to practice and are an example of an effective educator mechanism.

2. *Curricular mechanisms* are those challenges educators and administrators encounter when planning and implementing IPE. They include logistics, scheduling, shared outcomes, blending of program and course outcomes, accreditation requirements, and assessment.

The framework further defines mechanisms that influence how IPE and IPCP are implemented under the themes of institutional support mechanisms, working culture mechanisms, and environmental mechanisms.[5] These themes further describe the traits that stand as either enablers or barriers for educational institutions. However, it is important to note that these mechanisms are vital for both educational and clinical settings; when absent, they present as barriers to achieving IPE and IPCP.

Institutional Support Mechanisms

These mechanisms are vital to promoting a synergistic work setting and can shape a positive approach to collaboration.

- *Governance*—Includes support from the board of directors and an institutional commitment to an IPE or IPCP initiative.
- *Operational resources*—These include shared faculty models, shared course registrations, and shared administrative support.
- *Personnel policies*—These allow for flexibility and acceptance of less defined roles and responsibilities.
- *Supportive leadership*—Such leaders are willing to spend time and resources on a collaborative initiative and strategy.

Working Culture Mechanisms

Collaborative environments are supported when opportunities exist for shared governance and decision making.

- *Communication*—Should be routine and regular; shared opportunity allows for planning and decision making.
- *Conflict-resolution process*—Should be well defined as teams work though their process and procedures.
- *Shared decision making*—Difficulty can arise when one professional has more governance or decision making than another.

Environmental Mechanisms

Planned and focused space will promote collaborative practice; poorly planned space will deter collaboration.

- *Equipment and capital*—These include input from key stakeholders.
- *Facilities*—Should reflect collaboration versus hierarchy.
- *Space design*—Should eliminate barriers.

Most educational and health care institutions deal with one or more of these mechanisms in attempting to achieve IPE. Additionally, the suggestion that siloed departments may need to unbundle current policies, process, resources, and regulations to deliver IPE may appear to be an insurmountable charge. In the utopian model of IPE, this would be the goal, an unbundling of education as it has been delivered for hundreds of years. However, institutions and programs should not be

COLLABORATIVE CORNER
Professional Associations and IPE and IPCP

Vision 2025 of the American Occupational Therapy Association (AOTA) calls for interprofessional partnerships between disciplines. The American Speech-Language-Hearing Association (ASHA) road map for achieving its vision provides strategic objectives, one of which focuses on the advancement of IPE and IPCP in the preparation of students and ASHA professionals to work as members of a team across disciplines.

overwhelmed by the enormity of change and should instead focus on incremental changes leading to effective IPE delivery. One thing is certain: Health and education systems must work together, just as we expect professional disciplines to do, to develop the "collaborative practice-ready health workforce."[5(p7)]

History of IPCP

A historical review of resources and literature tends to provide a fragmented view of how IPCP and IPE have evolved. Because the history varies by region, country, and profession, only a brief history in the United States will be outlined here. This outline will focus first on the history of IPCP and then on IPE.

The traditional medical model that emerged at the beginning of the 1900s (figure 1.3) and has been the foundation of health care provision calls for a fee-for-service payment, largely recognizing providers for each singular service they provide and ignoring any payment for professionals working as a team or in a group. Fee-for-service payment fragmented care, and single-provider treatments have largely failed to keep up with the complex medical needs of society.[17]

The first formal effort to promote collaborative health care seems to be in the 1980s, when WHO endorsed the benefits of a team approach to care. Even as early as 1915, an article documented the team concept using a doctor, a social worker, and an educator working together to provide care. In 1920, the Dawson Report encouraged the team approach in the development of health centers, and during World War II, a multidisciplinary team approach was encouraged in the treatment of war injuries.[18]

Evidence of collaborative care in the United States became more notable in the era of managed care in the early 1990s, when professionals began to work in cooperation to provide medical care through third-party reimbursement. Some believed this would be the impetus to change the standard of care. Yet here we are today, with the majority of health care still being delivered and reimbursed by single professions and disciplines rather than as groups. The Patient Protection and Affordable Care Act of 2010 (ACA) additionally emphasizes that interprofessional teamwork is critical to successful patient-centered care. The ACA ties reimbursement to fiscal responsibility, patient outcomes, and quality. In theory, this legislation should promote new thinking around the way health care teams are organized and executed,

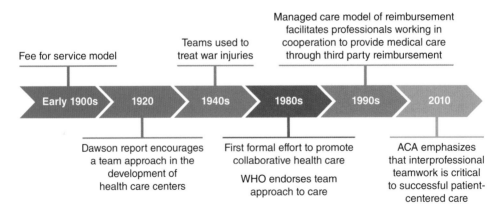

Figure 1.3   A history of collaboration in health care.

with a focus on value-based rather than volume-based care.[17] Although the ACA has been approved legislation since 2010, measurable outcomes are still being sought through pilot programs that have been implemented through the Centers for Medicare and Medicaid Services (CMS).[17,18]

The Institute for Healthcare Improvement (IHI) has proposed single points of treatment that are ineffective, and a more efficient model of health care should align with the Triple Aim (later developing into the Quadruple Aim), which is to improve the health of populations, improve the experience of care, and lower the cost. As a result, reimbursement models have responded, forcing providers to rethink the manner in which they provide care.[19,20]

There is no doubt that collaborative practice may hold some of the greatest promise for a seismic shift in health care. IPCP represents a paradigm shift away from uniprofessional health care and could conceivably change every aspect of delivery, reimbursement, education, and practice. Change in health care historically seems to be slow, but the previous steps do show promise of enabling mechanisms being implemented to promote change.

History of IPE

More than 100 years ago, a groundbreaking report challenged the system of educating health care professionals. The Flexner Report of 1910 made, among other recommendations, a commitment to the gold standard of medical education, the biomedical model. This reform of medical education might be considered the first step to standardizing medical education, but it also served to silo the educational system, compartmentalizing medical students from their health care peers.[6] It was not until the 1970s that support for a more team-based education began to emerge in the form of conferences and industry reports by the Institute of Medicine (IOM):

> The premise behind this team-based approach to medical education and practice is that health care delivered by well-functioning coordinated teams leads to better patient and family outcomes, more efficient health care services and a higher level of satisfaction among health care providers.[1(p2)]

Medical education in general has been described as generational, the first generation being a science-based curriculum and the second being a problem-based plan of study. The third, as it emerges, should take a systems approach by adopting IPE professional competencies.

The issue is not limited to the United States; a review of the interprofessional literature reveals hundreds of studies from all corners of the world, including South Africa, the United Kingdom, the United Arab Emirates, Germany, and Canada, to name just a few. Additionally, WHO has completed an international environmental scan that uncovered IPE efforts in 42 countries.[5]

Several initiatives have been instrumental in shaping IPE and IPCP and will continue to do so. Aside from the WHO framework, the Health Professions Accreditors Collaborative (HPAC) and the National Center for Interprofessional Practice and Education (NCIPE) released *Guidance on Developing Quality Interprofessional Education for the Health Professions*.[24] This work will undoubtedly help to guide educators and practitioners to a consensus regarding the development of quality projects and initiatives.

Though the history of IPE and IPCP is relatively new, the resources and organizations influencing the movement are many. New publications, conferences, and initiatives are offering numerous resources. Some of these are described here, while others are further explored in chapter 8.

Key Organizations and Resources

The following resources and organizations are referred to frequently in the literature and in reference to IPCP and IPE.

- *World Health Organization (WHO)*—Collaborative practice is indeed a global movement evidenced by the organizations and resources dedicated to the improvement of health care delivery. In 2010, WHO targeted key stakeholders in its Framework for Action on Interprofessional Education and Collaborative Practice. The proposed framework focuses on collaborative practice-ready health care workers and is referred to throughout this text as a landmark movement toward the ultimate goal of IPCP.

- *American Interprofessional Health Collaborative (AIHC)*—This collaborative is composed of individuals and organizations that transcend professional and organizational boundaries. AIHC promotes IPE, IPCP, and research that examines education–practice linkages between the two in order to improve health care delivery.[22]

- *Interprofessional Education Collaborative (IPEC)*—This collective focuses on the preparation of students and health care workers to "work in a collaborative practice model that is patient-centered, community-oriented and population-oriented, and interprofessional."[23] In 2009, 6 professional associations formed IPEC to prepare future clinicians in providing team-based care: the American Association of Colleges of Nursing (AACN), American Association of Colleges of Osteopathic Medicine (AACOM), American Association of Colleges of Pharmacy (AACP), American Dental Education Association (ADEA), American Association of Medical Colleges (AAMC), and Association of Schools and Programs of Public Health (ASPPH). Key to this work is the introduction of core competencies for IPE collaborative practice, including the following domains:

  - Values and ethics
  - Roles and responsibilities
  - Interprofessional communication
  - Teams and teamwork[23]

- *Institute for Healthcare Improvement (IHI)*—This organization has been partnering with leaders to think about ways to improve health care. In the early 1970s, IOM highlighted the importance of team-based patient care for safety and improved communication. The IHI Triple Aim initiative describes a framework that, via teamwork, will improve the patient experience of care, improve the health of populations, and reduce the cost of health care.

- *National Academy of Medicine (NAM)*—This association provides objective data and findings on matters pertinent to health care.

- *National Center for Interprofessional Practice and Education (NCIPE)*—This is the only U.S. organization designated by the Health Resources and Services Admin-

TOOLS OF IPE
Guiding Principles

In the landmark report on IPCP by the Robert Wood Johnson Foundation, a comparison and analysis of successful practices concluded that the following guiding principles were common to successful projects[21]:

- It takes time.
- Relationships matter.
- Pockets of interprofessional practice already exist.
- Name it—call it IPE or IPCP so people begin to recognize it.
- Start small.
- Creating a culture of interprofessional collaboration requires multiple reinforcing practices.

istration (HRSA) of the U.S. Department of Health and Human Services (HHS) as the center to provide leadership, scholarship, evidence, coordination, and national visibility to advance IPE and IPCP as a viable and efficient model for health care delivery.

• *Health Professions Accreditors Collaborative (HPAC)*—This group, founded in 2014 with only 6 accreditors, expanded membership to 25 accrediting bodies in 2019. HPAC was established to formulate communication across accrediting agencies with the goal of sharing information to coordinate change. A focus of the collaborative is removing barriers to IPE to advance the Quadruple Aim through a document titled *Guidance on Developing Quality Interprofessional Education for the Health Professions*.

• *National Collaborative for Improving the Clinical Learning Environment (NCICLE)*—This organization is a unique public–private partnership providing leadership, evidence, and resources to guide people on the use of IPE and collaborative practice to enhance the experience of health care, improve population health, and reduce the overall cost of care. NEXUS conference is an annual collaboration of leaders in IPE.[26]

Summary

To achieve a health care culture where continuous care (versus episodic encounters) is the standard, health care professionals must work in collaboration and not in isolation. As such, educational transformation is needed. The framework for need has been set in chapter 1 with an outline of key terminologies. A large body of evidence supports the rationale for transformational change in health care and education. Historical evidence outlines the beginning of this transformation, but there is still much work to be done. Many organizations and agencies have begun to address the need for sustainable change, and perhaps if they all collaborate, the possibility for success exists. The following chapters will present a comprehensive approach to IPE and IPCP, as well as strategies to support sustainability and change.

The next chapter introduces models of IPE delivery in the academic setting. Looking ahead, chapters 2, 3, and 4 focus on IPE in academic settings, including the evidence supporting its use. Chapters 5, 6, and 7 look at IPCP in the health care setting. Finally, chapter 8 focuses on the sustainability of both IPE and IPCP initiatives and programs.

CASE STUDY Debriefing

In the days since Russell's passing, the professionals involved in his care have asked themselves what they could have done differently. They have questioned how they could have integrated their discipline-specific roles to improve the delivery of care. For example, the nurses, SLP, and OT were all concerned with the safety of Russell's feeding and swallowing but only looked at the issue from their unique perspectives. Had the team worked together, the outcome might have been very different. One potential scenario suggests that the team would have met or communicated before the weekend, when fewer health care providers would be available. They might have suggested that Russell should not be left alone or only with family during any eating activity or that unsupervised oral feedings should not be allowed. Or they might have suggested a team meeting with the family to teach precautions for swallowing. One thing is perfectly clear: Better communication could have potentially prevented this fatal scenario.

Many enabling factors were present but not embraced. Most important may have been the missed IPCP opportunity to solve a complex problem. Barriers also existed, such as silos, fragmented charting with EMR systems, and the varying terminologies used among health professionals. As you discuss the case of Russell, continue to think about both enablers and barriers in an approach to remediating such tragedies. Consider other resources and evidence to support the change. What changes in the workplace are needed?

Case Study Discussion Questions

1. What role could professionals from each discipline have played? What role should the team have played?
2. What could have been done differently to better support Russell? His family?
3. How might the family have been more engaged in Russell's care?
4. What solutions might have resulted if the professionals collaborated prior to the weekend events?
5. What changes specific to communication can be implemented to prevent a future tragedy at this facility?
6. How might the facility leaders facilitate better collaboration and communication?
7. What are some first steps the facility could take to facilitate a more collaborative approach?
8. Who might serve as champions or leaders in supporting a collaborative approach to care in this facility?
9. What types of changes in the space, facility, or process could facilitate a collaborative change?

Models of Delivery

Joy Doll, OTD, OTR/L
Anthony Breitbach, PhD, ATC, FASAHP
Kathrin Eliot, PhD, RD, FAND

Objectives

After reading this chapter, the reader will be able to do the following:

- Incorporate essential knowledge, skills, and abilities into an IPE curriculum.
- Design learning objectives or outcomes that engage in reflection and building skills for interprofessional teamwork.
- Design IPE curriculum that reflects the IPEC core competencies.
- Use Kirkpatrick's expanded outcomes typology to guide assessment of the IPEC core competencies.

CASE STUDY New City University

Administrators of New City University have charged a faculty committee with developing an IPE program. For the past 5 years, faculty members from 3 health professions have worked on grassroots efforts to initiate IPE activities. Faculty members have been driven by their passion for improving education and practice through collaboration. They have enjoyed learning about, from, and with each other while delving into new areas of teaching and practice. However, IPE accreditation mandates have forced this group to become more formalized and to decide how to implement IPE at an institutional level.

Dr. Lusky from the nursing program wants to start from the ground up. He is the director of the undergraduate program and believes that entry-level IPE will make the greatest impact on students and programs. From what he has read in the literature, engaging students in IPE before their professional identities are ingrained allows them to be more open to working with others. He believes this foundation is necessary to create buy-in from the other programs not currently involved in IPE activities.

(continued)

Case Study *(continued)*

Conversely, Dr. Simons from the graduate program in physical therapy (PT) wants to develop an initiative at the graduate level. She believes the maximum impact will come from working with students in the clinical phase of their education, because there are more students from a greater number of programs learning together in the clinical phase. The dean of the College of Health Sciences, in which Dr. Simons' program resides, has put pressure on her to deliver more IPE opportunities to the graduate programs.

Many competing interests and outside pressures are starting to press on the strong foundation this group has established. Similarly, faculty members from programs who were not engaged at the grassroots level are displaying varying degrees of interest. For example, the representative from the audiology program has repeatedly stated that the program is not interested in participating in what faculty see as an additional burden to students and curriculum.

Two groups seem to be developing around the polarities of a more didactic undergraduate program and a more clinically integrated postbaccalaureate program. The provost and deans insist that IPE offerings must be available to all programs, but all programs do not have to participate in every learning experience. The administration notifies the faculty committee that an IPE proposal is due by the end of the academic year. With dissenting attitudes, pressures from the administration, logistical barriers, and varying accreditation needs, how can this committee work as a team to move the initiative forward to create an effective IPE model of delivery at New City University?

IPE has been identified by WHO as occurring when students from two or more professions "learn about, from, and with each other to enable effective collaboration and improve health outcomes."[1(p13)] Although this definition appears to be fairly simple, implementing IPE is anything but. Due to historical precedence, accreditation guidelines, and cultural norms in health professions, IPE requires the educator to be creative and focus not only on pedagogy but also on negotiating a culture change in the delivery of health care education. Traditionally, health care education has focused on forming students into professionals, less so on preparing them to collaborate and engage in teamwork with other health professionals.[1] In today's health care education, many institutions recognize the value of moving beyond simply teaching profession-centric **cognitive skills** and preparing graduates with **affective skills** to be ready to collaborate as part of a health care team.[2] Health care organizations have called on educational institutions to prepare health professions students to work in teams, the intent of IPE.[2]

IPE and IPCP are an evolving field. With the goal of IPE being the development of team-ready health care practitioners, educators must recognize that developing a team presents the essential challenge of integrating a distinct set of abilities and roles to create a cohesive effort.[9] This chapter summarizes the theoretical basis of IPE. Theoretical approaches are followed by recognition of the multiple modes of delivery that are based on the delivery context (e.g., academic institution, clinical

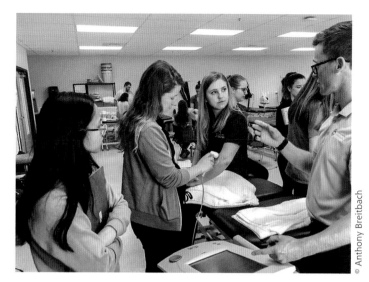

© Anthony Breitbach

Peer teaching between health professional students.

learning environment). Lastly, assessment of the learner across multiple environments and through a diversity of interprofessional pedagogical models will be addressed.

Theoretical Approaches

IPE should be designed with an evidence-based approach using theory, including both established theoretical approaches and heuristic approaches. Multiple theoretical approaches exist that provide guidance in developing IPE curricula. IPE curricula should ensure that all IPE activities align with appropriate and relevant theoretical approaches.

Educational Theory

According to Oandasan and Reeves,[3] educational theory—including adult learning theory, problem-based learning, and experiential learning—provides the basis for all IPE. For learners to develop team skills for IPCP, they need the opportunity to practice and engage in interprofessional experiences. IPE experiences should be designed on a robust and relevant theoretical basis. Educators should discern which theoretical approach matches their IPE curriculum. According to HPAC's *Guidance on Developing Quality Interprofessional Education for the Health Professions*, an IPE curriculum should include the following: rationale, outcome-based goals, deliberate design, and assessment and evaluation. Although no specific theories are mentioned in the document, the recommendation of a rationale ensures educators consider appropriate educational theory as applied to IPE.[4]

Kolb's Theory of Experiential Learning

In Kolb's theory of experiential learning, the intent is to bring together learners to engage in a process of thinking, doing, and reflecting. Structuring interprofessional learning activities following Kolb's work provides a theoretical basis for structuring meaningful and relevant experiences. Kolb's theory is considered an adult learning theory and has been defined as an "experiential conflict-filled process out of which the development of insight, understanding and skills comes."[5(p5)] The key components of Kolb's theory include learners' active engagement in understanding the meaning of phenomena, reflecting, and integrating new knowledge with previous knowledge. It is a cyclical process that mirrors the values of IPE, which require practice and engagement to evolve in interprofessional skills. In Kolb's learning cycle, learners engage in a process of active experimentation (planning), concrete experience (doing a learning activity), reflective observation, and abstract conceptualization (learning from experience). This cycle is repeated as one learns and engages. It is a grounding theoretical framework for IPE experiences that are framed using the Kolb learning cycle.[6]

Situated Learning

Interprofessional encounters vary based on patient needs. Due to the diversity of health care teams based on individual patients, educators must design IPE using situated learning. Situated learning is "scenario-based learning embedded within a particular social and physical environment."[7(p175)] IPE curricula should recognize that the social and physical environments will vary based on the learners, the health care environment, and the patient and family involved. Situated learning theory notes that every IPE encounter will vary based on the cultural, social, and physical context. Educators should recognize that situated learning provides a foundation to recognize the complexity of interprofessional interactions.

Cs of Teamwork

Infusing educational theory with concepts of team-based theory provides a strong base for IPE. Based on the evidence and literature on teams both inside and outside health care, Salas and colleagues developed a heuristic model based on the knowledge, skills, and attitudes needed for successful health care teamwork (figure 2.1).[8,74] Salas and colleagues recommended designing IPE that uses the Cs to help develop team skills in learners.[8,74]

Foundation of IPE Teaching and Learning

Scanning the literature on IPE and IPCP quickly reveals that diversity and context dictate the methods of delivery, whether in the academic or clinical environment. IPE and IPCP are not delivered in a one-size-fits-all approach; rather, they challenge educators to consider the learning environment, learning outcomes, and delivery context. For example, in the case study at the beginning of the chapter, IPE was accomplished by faculty champions passionate about the approach, but a clear plan was not in place when institutional support for IPE expanded. However, examples of best practice exist at many academic and clinical institutions. Chapter 1 lends

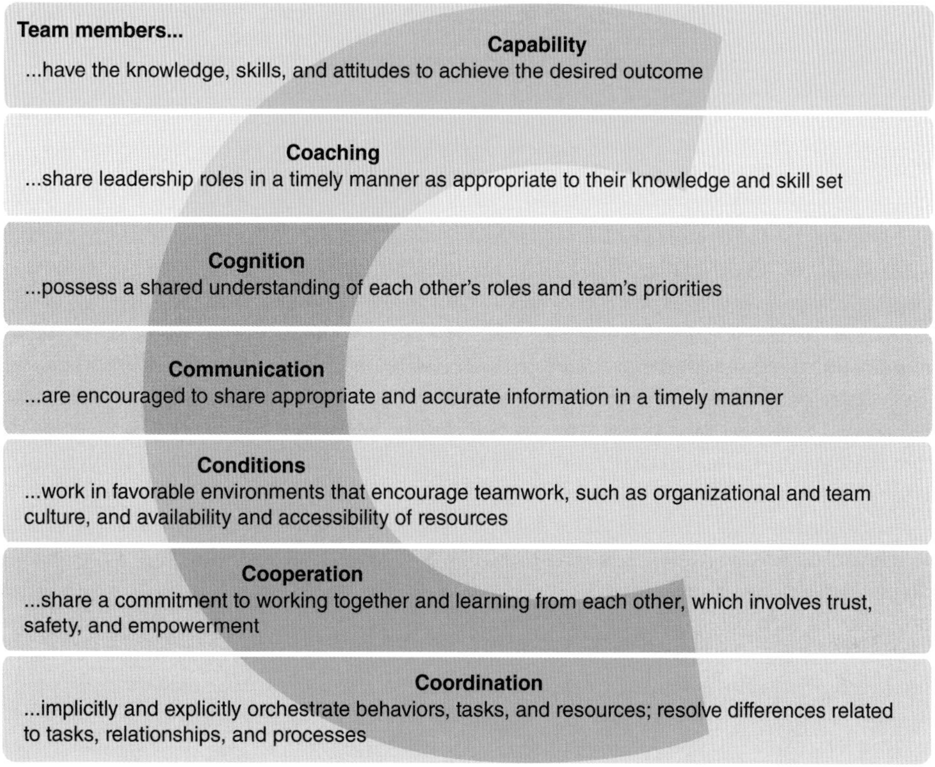

Team members...   **Capability**
...have the knowledge, skills, and attitudes to achieve the desired outcome

Coaching
...share leadership roles in a timely manner as appropriate to their knowledge and skill set

Cognition
...possess a shared understanding of each other's roles and team's priorities

Communication
...are encouraged to share appropriate and accurate information in a timely manner

Conditions
...work in favorable environments that encourage teamwork, such as organizational and team culture, and availability and accessibility of resources

Cooperation
...share a commitment to working together and learning from each other, which involves trust, safety, and empowerment

Coordination
...implicitly and explicitly orchestrate behaviors, tasks, and resources; resolve differences related to tasks, relationships, and processes

Figure 2.1   Cs of teamwork.

credibility to IPCP regarding benefits to systems, procedures, and health outcomes; however, there remains a gap in the research on how IPE should be implemented.[10] Although the lack of a clear road map results in a challenging ambiguity, that same ambiguity offers extensive opportunity to innovate and engage in creative approaches to advance both IPE and IPCP.

As discussed by Masten and colleagues, the road map to IPE is more about implementing culture change than simply taking an educational approach.[11] It requires leaders and educators to consider cultural context as a driver for the design and implementation of IPE, which has been presented as a best practice and a deliberate design approach.[4] Masten and colleagues describe these cultural changes following 5 stages (figure 2.2):

- *Stage 1: Awakening*—The process of recognizing the value and importance of IPE begins.
- *Stage 2: Giving lip service*—Leaders and educators move beyond talking about IPE to implementing structures to support it, like faculty time and reward.
- *Stage 3: Parallel play*—Pockets of IPE exist but are often not institutionalized.
- *Stage 4: Group play*—IPE curriculum advances, with administrators recognizing the challenges and faculty champions receiving support to move IPE forward.
- *Stage 5: Cultural transformation*—IPE is being implemented well and is recognized by the wider university.[11]

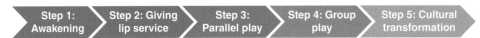

Figure 2.2   Stages of IPE development.

This approach provides a road map for the stages of cultural transformation necessary to make IPE a sustained reality (for more on sustainability, see chapter 8). Despite the lack of clear evidence for an ideal IPE curriculum, the literature on teamwork and team science provides extensive support to pedagogical approaches. The reality remains that attitudes, behaviors, and skills that elicit successful IPCP do not require a clear end point of accomplishment or competence; rather, they require educators to prepare students for an ambiguous and unclear journey.[13] This chapter provides a foundation to prepare learners (e.g., students, residents, fellows, clinicians, faculty) to gain the attitudes, behaviors, and skills to negotiate the contemporary health care landscape that is keenly focused on population health and societal needs.

Another challenge to educators in IPE is that many of the skills required for effective teamwork require learners to engage in activities that promote self-awareness, respect for others, conflict engagement, and effective team communication.[1] In addition, health care professionals have traditionally experienced discomfort with some of the skills required to be an effective team member.[13] Educators themselves might not be comfortable facilitating these topics, either. Furthermore, professional development for faculty takes mostly a self-study approach and is developed through faculty champions passionate about interprofessionalism.[14] Seeking professional development and a clear faculty development plan on IPE topics should be part of any program (see chapter 3 for more on professional development models). The learners here are not only the students but also the faculty who are teaching and role modeling interprofessional concepts.[15] Resources for faculty development are available through NCIPE and through AIHC, the professional association for IPE.

Many IPCP skills and abilities require individual skill building and awareness of one's own strengths and weaknesses. This perspective is emphasized in the IPEC core competencies for IPCP (figure 2.3), which include the following[12]:

- *Values and ethics for interprofessional practice*—Work with individuals from other professions to maintain a climate of mutual respect and shared values.

- *Roles and responsibilities*—Use the knowledge of one's own role and of other professions to assess and address the health care needs of patients and to promote and advance the health of populations.

- *Interprofessional communication*—Communicate with patients, families, communities, and professionals in health and other fields in a responsive and responsible manner that supports a team approach to the promotion and maintenance of health and the prevention and treatment of disease.

- *Teams and teamwork*—Apply relationship-building values and the principles of team dynamics to perform effectively in various team roles to plan, deliver, and evaluate patient-centered care and population health programs and policies that are safe, timely, efficient, effective, and equitable.

Reprinted by permission from Association of American Medical Colleges, on behalf of IPEC.

Each competency has subcompetencies that provide guidance for interprofessional skill development. Engaging students in IPE activities that allow them to practice being part of a team (and to begin to maneuver the challenges of teamwork) is critical to meeting the learning outcomes of IPE. As identified by Clark, a range of tools can be used to develop awareness of both one's self and other team members that can help promote collaboration[16]:

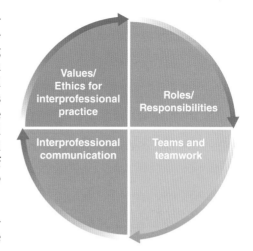

Figure 2.3 IPEC core competencies.

- *Myers–Briggs Type Indicator*—Identifies how one prefers to make decisions.
- *StrengthsFinder*—Identifies one's natural talents.
- *Kolb Learning Style Inventory*—Identifies one's preferred learning style.
- *DiSC*—Identifies one's personal style.

Being aware of one's own perspective and learning the roles and responsibilities of others, as guided by the core competencies, should be the premise of all IPE.

Learning Strategies

Studies have identified a breadth and depth of IPE across institutions. The diversity of length, team composition, and learning experiences makes it challenging to identify an exact road map for ideal IPE experiences.[17,18] HPAC set the stage for quality IPE by highlighting the principles of adult learning, allowing participants time for engagement to understand diverse perspectives and activities that afford an exchange of information between participants.[4] In addition, the variety of accreditation requirements for IPE establish both challenges and opportunities.[19] Despite these challenges, several strategies have been shown to be critical to student learning in IPE: engaging in reflection, building skills for engaging in teams, and establishing learning objectives or outcomes.

Focus on teamwork and team science has emphasized that health professionals need a variety of skills to ensure successful collaboration. As previously stated, understanding teams and teamwork is a core competency.[12] In IPCP, it is expected that health professionals understand team development, share accountability, and reflect upon team performance.

Various factors have been noted in high-performing health care teams. Some of these are supported by the context in which the team functions, including time for teamwork and leadership that supports teamwork.[20] As noted by Sargeant and colleagues, "Effective collaborative healthcare teams share common goals, understand each other's roles, demonstrate respect for each other, use clear communication, resolve conflict effectively, and are flexible."[21(p229)] At the same time, skill building by individuals is important to ensure team success, which is where IPE can play a role in shaping today's health care. Effective health care teams have been documented as made up of individuals who demonstrate the knowledge, skills, and attitude to collaborate.[22] High-performing health care teams include members who have a shared understanding of how to work together, hold a desire to work together, and engage in humility to cooperate and compromise.[23] Recognizing these identified skills, educators and IPE facilitators must create a learning experience focused on building teaming skills among a variety of health professions (for more on teaming, see chapter 6). Furthermore, the core competencies provide a framework for developing any IPE curriculum.

Reflection

As with any pedagogical approach, IPE is guided by best practices in delivery and engagement. Although there is not a single approach that stands out as the best practice, certain elements have been identified as critical to providing quality IPE in academic environments. Because IPE is ridden with challenges for learners grappling with their own professional identity (and how it emerges on a team), reflection is a skill that helps both the individual learner and the team. As Oandasan and Reeves point out, IPE is a swampy area of learning where "students must grapple with a number of complex issues related to hierarchy, role blurring, leadership, decision-making, communication, respect—to name but a few."[3(p26)] A critical skill necessary for developing self-awareness, engaging in difficult conversations, and not shying away from conflict on teams is reflection. Reflection is well defined by John Dewey as "active, persistent and careful consideration of any belief or supposed form of knowledge in the light of the grounds that support it and the further conclusion to which it tends."[24(p9)]

Similar to IPE, a best practice (method or structure) for reflection has yet to be identified. Instead, reflection method and type should be defined and vetted by the educator based on the learners involved and the activity. Learners can benefit from a framework for reflection, such as the "What? So what? Now what?" format (see the Collaborative Corner sidebar). Reflection is a useful pedagogy for enhancing many learning experiences, including case analysis, community experience, simulation, and clinical learning experience. In addition, reflection can be implemented verbally in a briefing or debriefing or in written form using activities such as journaling or reflection papers.[14] The type of reflection used matters less than ensuring it is a learning process infused in IPE. Educators should consider the type of activity being conducted and which type of reflection is appropriate for the team. It is important to remember that reflection without intention (or that is not evaluated) does not offer value. In order to build the skills necessary to prepare collaboration-ready learners, reflection should be facilitated or participants should receive feedback on the process to help them grow in their ability for reflection. The overall intent is to make reflection a practice that can aid in both professional and team growth, fostering a dual identity.

COLLABORATIVE CORNER
What? So What? Now What?

Use the following as a guide to the "What? So what? Now what?" format for completing reflection papers.

What?

Document the experience and what happened. What did you do in the specific session or encounter?

So What?

Describe the aspects of the event that affected you and why. What foundational behaviors applied here? What was or will be the impact on the patient? What were your experiences, attitudes, or emotions regarding the project?

Now What?

Apply your experience to your future clinical practice. How will you incorporate this experience into your future actions? Did it help you identify any insights into experiences you are having during clinical rotations? How may this event inform your knowledge, attitudes, and behaviors as a developing clinician? How did this experience help you identify anything you would like to learn or do going forward as a clinician?

A common IPE activity is gathering participants around a case study to analyze process and outcomes. The learners may share roles and responsibilities and develop a collaborative care plan for the patient. These cases tend to be complex and offer opportunities for multiple professions to engage with the patient. In these types of activities, engaging students at the end in a reflection on the experience of collaboration can provide a valuable learning opportunity. Here are examples of questions for reflection following a case analysis:

- What was the most difficult part of working together as an interprofessional team?
- What would have made your experience as part of an interprofessional team better?
- Describe what you learned from this experience about yourself and your profession.
- Describe what you learned about other professions.
- Why do you think IPCP is important in today's health care environment?
- What have you learned from this activity that you will use in practice?

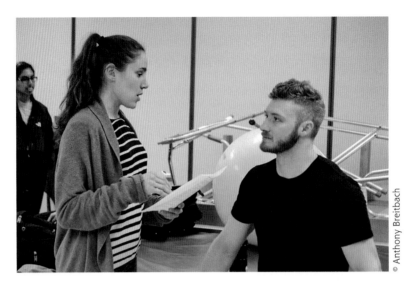

Role-play between students.

Briefs and debriefs are structures for reflection and communication that can be implemented in a variety of IPE activities and are often strategies used in clinical practice. **Briefing** and **debriefing** can facilitate reflection without significant challenges to implementation. These are strategic approaches provided in **TeamSTEPPS**, evidence-based modules developed with the goal of optimizing patient outcomes through improved communication and teamwork.[25] Examples and resources for TeamSTEPPS, including briefs and debriefs, are available through the Agency for Healthcare Research and Quality (AHRQ).[26]

A **brief** is a short, intentional gathering of multiple health care professionals before an experience to establish the plan and next steps. Members may do quick introductions and then discuss a collaborative approach. Briefs can set the tone for the experience and help learners feel more comfortable engaging with learners outside their profession, which is necessary for effective health care teams. Debriefs offer a strategy for postactivity reflection where the team reflects on what went well in the experience and what could go better the next time. Brief and debrief questions can vary based on experience but should be intentional and include a member to facilitate the experience. In addition, because reflection requires practice and skill building, feedback should be provided to both individual members and to the team about their ability to reflect.[27] As Clark identifies, the space, place, and time for reflection are important for it to become a practice that teams engage in for IPE as well as for teamwork in the health care setting.[16]

Learning Objectives and Learning Outcomes

All IPE experiences should have clear learning objectives and outcomes that apply to all learners engaged in the experience. Educators from multiple professions should discern the best objectives for each activity. IPEC's *Core Competencies for Interprofessional Collaborative Practice* acts as a guiding document to develop these learning objectives.[12] One strategy is to assign a learning objective from an IPE activity in each core competency: teams and teamwork, interprofessional communication, values and ethics, and roles and responsibilities. The subcompetencies under each core competency delineate more detailed focal points and provide a foundation for learning objectives. Learning objectives and outcomes can also be applied to a broader IPE curriculum.[12] Gunaldo and colleagues performed such an exercise that is a great exemplar of how the core competencies can guide the development of meaningful learning outcomes.[28]

Critical to aligning with learning objectives and outcomes is pairing with an effective assessment to measure whether learners have mastered the targeted skill in IPE activities.[29] Assessment of IPE has emerged with its own opportunities and challenges. The IOM, now known as NAM, published an interprofessional learning continuum in 2015 to provide a comprehensive perspective on the continuum of learning in IPE to help educators consider the complexities and opportunities of IPE and team-based care (figure 2.4).[30]

Although assessment remains a challenge, some guidance can be sought from the Kirkpatrick model, which was applied to the interprofessional learning continuum.[24] The Kirkpatrick model has been used as an evaluation framework for IPE across the literature. The model came about in the 1960s as a method to advance learning and assessment as learners evolve. In addition to IPE, it has also been adopted in medical research.[31]

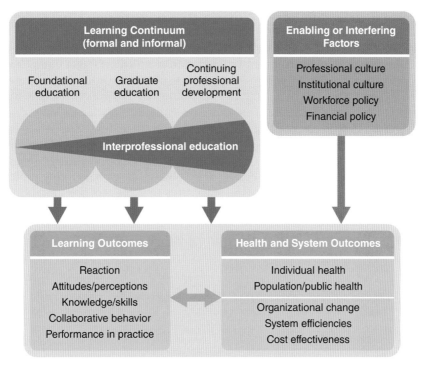

Figure 2.4 Interprofessional learning continuum model.

Institute of Medicine. 2015. Measuring the Impact of Interprofessional Education on Collaborative Practice and Patient Outcomes. https://doi.org/10.17226/21726. Reprinted with permission from the National Academy of Sciences, Courtesy of the National Academies Press, Washington, D.C.

The Kirkpatrick model identifies levels of learning assessment that can provide guidance for designing learning objectives and outcomes to match (see chapter 3 for an examination of the model related to assessing IPE and IPCP). In the Kirkpatrick model, assessment is viewed in levels beginning with reaction and moving through attitudes and perceptions, knowledge and skills, collaborative behavior, and performance in practice. Learning outcomes and learning objectives should be measured based on the level of the experience; early learners (prelicense) may focus on lower levels (1-2), while late learners (postlicense) focus on higher levels (3-4).[30] The key is to match the learner's level (prelicense to postlicense) with the right experience, alongside an assessment with a valid and reliable tool that matches both the Kirkpatrick level and the IPE pedagogy.[32] In addition, academic programs and hospital departments may assess the effectiveness of IPE and IPCP with the intent to share with and compare across programs and departments; this approach has been suggested to offer a more efficient and rigorous evaluation of IPE and IPCP outcomes.[30] NCIPE has a repository of assessment tools that can be a resource for faculty wanting to assess the learner experience. Ultimately, educators and facilitators of professional development in IPE need to explore available tools to accurately assess learner outcomes.

Team-Based Skills

Learners need the opportunity to address long-engrained hierarchies, beliefs, and biases about health care professions. Due to traditions and belief systems long institutionalized in both health care education and practice, learners must feel comfortable challenging implicit bias and hierarchies that often lead to conflict in health care teams.[33] Additionally, many health care providers entered their fields to care for others and feel reticent to engage in conflict.[13] IPE can equip learners with the skills necessary to engage in teams in an effective, productive manner. But addressing hierarchy, bias, and conflict are not innate skills, and learners need to experience teamwork to be able to use these strategies in clinical practice. Educators must consider how to employ IPE learning activities that allow students to engage in the difficult conversations necessary to build skills for health care teamwork. Without careful consideration of these dynamics and the opportunity to engage in fruitful discussion and learning activities involving these challenging topics, IPE activities are at risk of reinforcing the structures that prevent collaboration.[34] IPE activities that do not recognize these dynamics do not adequately prepare learners for the challenges they will encounter in team-based health care.[28]

The literature clearly shows that teams function most effectively when psychological safety has been nurtured. Psychological safety occurs when team members can speak and engage with others without fear of retaliation,[35] when a climate of trust is established among team members. In most cases, psychological safety can only be cultivated in long-term teams where members consistently engage in IPE together.[36] Educators should ensure that IPE activities allow learners the opportunity to engage in teams across time in order to experience team development and the skills required for a high-performing team.

Modes of Instruction

The application of educational theory to IPE is relevant across the IPE learning continuum for learners, facilitators, and administrators.[37,38] Currently, there does not appear to be a widely accepted theoretical underpinning for the curricular implementation of IPE across any contexts. However, scholars have attempted to determine the most applicable theories and evaluate their appropriateness for IPE and IPCP. Kolb's theory of experiential learning shows promise as a model to support students learning to collaborate.[39] Research has examined the applicability of this theory in a case study approach and found it to have great potential to create change in cognition in students working through the concrete process of collaboration.

Educational theories within the context of IPE focus on 3 theories: theory of social capital, adult learning theory, and the sociological perspective.[40] Additionally, the importance of adult learning theory is underscored by Hammick and colleagues in their review of IPE literature, suggesting that principles from this theory promote a positive reception of IPE in learners.[40] Each of these theories shows promise in contributing toward a better understanding of how IPE incorporates into curricula across the education continuum; identifying theories to apply to IPE continues to be an important charge. Solid application of theory helps to inform teaching pedagogy. Additionally, theories can better equip educators to engage students in their own understanding and appreciation of IPE.[41]

Regardless of the theoretical underpinning, format, or structure of IPE programming, the goal should be to develop future practitioners who are prepared to be collaborative, reflective members of an interprofessional health care team. A solid IPE foundation should encourage students to think critically and assess their own learning and performance.[18] This can be achieved in a combination of delivery models, including in-person learning, collaborative online learning, and experiential learning (figure 2.5; see the sidebar IPE Learning Modalities).

In-Person Learning

Didactic instruction is the cornerstone of the development of IPE skills. Topics for didactic instruction for early learners should focus on basic teamwork and collaboration skills.[35] In-person, synchronous IPE pedagogy ranges from brief workshops (2 hours to 1 day) to semester or yearlong coursework. Face-to-face interventions as short as a few hours can be effective in changing attitudes toward other professions' roles and responsibilities, but program designers should carefully consider where

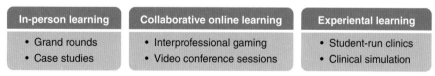

Figure 2.5 IPE learning modalities.

IPE LEARNING MODALITIES

In-Person Learning

In-person learning involves face-to-face, synchronous activities where students or clinicians from one health profession learn with, about, and from students or clinicians from another health profession. Examples include the following:

- Large-scale lectures or discussions
- Faculty-facilitated team meetings
- Grand rounds or case discussions
- Clinical observations

Collaborative Online Learning

In online collaborative learning activities, completed synchronously or asynchronously, students or clinicians from one health profession learn with, about, and from students or clinicians from another health profession. Examples include the following:

- Video conference discussions
- Mock EMR collaborations
- Interprofessional gaming
- Chat room discussions
- Clinical simulations
- Telehealth teams

Experiential Learning

Experiential learning activities provide opportunities for students or clinicians from one health profession to learn with, about, and from students or clinicians from another health profession in real-world or simulated activities. Examples include the following:

- Clinical rotations
- Standardized patients
- Clinical simulations
- Service learning
- Case competitions
- Student-run clinics

Adapted from Health Professions Accreditors Collaborative, *Guidance on Developing Quality Interprofessional Education for the Health Professions* (Chicago, IL: Health Professions Accreditors Collaborative, 2019).

TOOLS OF IPE
Impact of Team Composition on Student Perceptions

A longitudinal example of factors that affect teamwork as explored by Lairamore and colleagues shows the benefits of intentional team development when using case-based IPE in preparing students for collaborative practice.[42] In their work, 6 cohorts of students participated in discussions on either broad or targeted case scenarios. The data, collected over 6 years, showed participants' improvement in readiness for interprofessional learning and interdisciplinary education perceptions. Furthermore, the cohorts were categorized as smaller (5 health professions) or larger (10 health professions), and, interestingly, the smaller cohorts exhibited a greater impact on the students' perceptions of teamwork. Therefore, when planning groups for IPE activities, faculty need to consider the optimal size and number of professions, recognizing that more is not always necessarily better.

to place these experiences in the curriculum.[36] The mix of professions, learners' previous IPE experiences, and expectations for learning outcomes will influence the ideal placement of these sessions to maximize their effectiveness.

In a face-to-face setting, many factors are important to successful interactions that build teamwork skills. For example, size and layout of the space chosen for the interactions should be carefully planned to maximize comfortable exchange of ideas among team members. Faculty facilitators who can help small teams engage in activities and reflection are also important to ensure a positive learning experience. In addition, educators should consider the types and levels of learners to ensure the experience is beneficial for all. Face-to-face IPE often requires educators to not only deliver content but also coordinate many logistics around both students and faculty peers who assist with the instruction.

Collaborative Online Learning

One of the challenges frequently reported in the IPE literature is the incredible demand on time and space to bring learners from multiple programs into a face-to-face environment.[43,44] Additionally, some professions, such as dietetics and athletic training, may not be physically located in a college or campus with other health professions, thus providing additional challenges to in-person pedagogy.[45] In this case, online learning, whether synchronous or asynchronous, can meet the needs of both faculty and learners. Online learning releases the burden of finding time and space for multiple learners across several professions. Remote learning may also allow for flexibility among learning styles and preferences for students.[46]

Delivery of remote IPE will look different for individual programs based on their goals and desired outcomes but may include elements such as building virtual communities where students can engage in the treatment of simulated patients.

Other options include online learning groups, group chats, and virtual interactive patients.[47]

One consideration for remote learning is the increased demand for technology on behalf of both facilitators and learners. Both faculty and students need to be proficient in using the technology required to engage in distance learning, which may necessitate additional training and resources. Specifically, facilitators must be prepared to effectively engage students in a virtual environment.[48] Additionally, they should acknowledge the potential for learners to become isolated in a virtual environment and take care to engage students in ways that foster interaction. A potential solution to prevent isolation is to provide a hybrid model where some instruction is provided in person as opposed to entirely online.[49] One of the authors provides a foundational IPE course online that is self-paced and based on competencies. Although learners appreciate the flexibility, many report disappointment at the lack of interactivity. Educators have to balance logistics with pedagogical practices when determining IPE delivery. Consider the challenges and opportunities of each mode of instruction as you build an IPE plan (table 2.1).

Experiential Learning

Experiential learning is critical to developing the collaboration skills required for IPCP to become a reality. There are myriad options for implementing experiential learning, from the simple (case-based learning) to the complex (high-fidelity simulation). These methods encourage students to explore their own roles as well as those of their peers and provide opportunities to practice various communication techniques. Case-based learning (CBL) is enjoyable for both instructors and students and can be implemented either in person or online. If conducted in small groups, CBL helps to engage each learner more deeply.[50]

Table 2.1 Challenges and Opportunities With Modes of Instruction

Type of Instruction	Challenges	Opportunities
In-person learning	Scheduling Room size	Active engagement of learners in one time and place
Collaborative online learning	Limited opportunity for interactivity	Opportunities for many learners to engage
		Delivery without concern about student scheduling or location
		Multiple locations to collaborate with a shared purpose
Experiential learning, on-site development	Access to community partners or simulation facilities	Opportunities to practice in an active learning environment

Simulation remains a popular method for practicing interprofessional skills. A common and effective simulation is the use of a standardized patient. Standardized patients are actors who have been trained to simulate patients with conditions and situations determined by the facilitators. A critical component of an effective simulation is the debriefing process. Whether conducted in person or remotely, facilitators should be trained to conduct effective debriefing sessions. Often, this process is enhanced when two or more IPE facilitators from different professions conduct the debriefing.

At one of the author's institutions, a competition in health care error simulation occurs twice a year. Not only is the simulation engaging, it allows students to collaborate and reflect on the value of a team in a health care situation.[50] The simulation requires writing a new case each year, along with scheduling the simulation facility. The nursing department generously supports this activity by allowing use of their simulation room and resources. IPE educators not well versed in simulation can partner with a simulation center to offer these activities.

Models of Delivery

IPE is delivered in many formats and many contexts. Instructors and staff need to examine their level of administrative commitment, availability of resources, mix and level of health professional programs, and curricular flexibility as they develop their own best-fit model. Table 2.2 presents an interprofessional pedagogy matrix that suggests how IPE programs accommodate these factors.[51]

Table 2.2   Interprofessional Pedagogy Matrix

Time and Resource Demands	Intracurricular (internal or integrated into formal academic curricula)	Extracurricular (outside of formal academic curricula)
Low	IPE competencies included in individual program courses	One-time interprofessional workshop or orientation
	IPE modules embedded in individual program courses	Interprofessional grand rounds observations
	Cross-listed courses with IPE content	Interprofessional simulation activities
Medium	Single IPE introductory course	Regularly scheduled seminars, workshops, and so on
	Multiple IPE core content courses	Interprofessional capstone projects, portfolios, and so on
	Academic curriculum including practicum	Mentored interprofessional service learning activities
High	Academic concentration, major or minor	Established clinical practice using IPCP teams

Introductory IPE Experiences (Early Learners, Kirkpatrick Levels 1-2)

Regardless of context, most IPE programs have some sort of introductory learning experience. This lays a foundation for the more contextually relevant activities that follow.[52] These experiences vary by the context and professional mix of the academic units.

The primary themes of these activities usually cluster around the IPEC competency domains,[12] the Quadruple Aim,[20] and skill sets common to all health professions. These common skills could include professionalism, evidence-based practice, ethics, health literacy, advocacy, conflict management, and communication. The teaching format varies widely depending on the academic programs involved, their respective accreditation standards, the mission and structure of the academic institutions, and the needs of the students.

A challenge present in most introductory IPE experiences is scale. Universities and colleges want this type of experience to be a common component of all their programs for health professions. IPE faculty members need to address this scale in their instructional design. When multiple programs are engaged, the demand can easily grow to more than 500 students in an academic year.

One method of teaching an introductory experience is large, face-to-face didactic sessions that leverage technology and administrative support to enhance the course delivery by a teaching team of several faculty members. In this type of model, students are placed in teams who sit in class together and cocreate team assignments in class based on the content presented in the session. This type of course emphasizes intentional design and preparation that enable organic learning in class sessions. In this model, students are required to individually do readings outside of class on content that they will apply in their team activities. It also includes an introductory activity where members get to know each other and lay down team principles regarding processes. The course culminates in a team project of a public service announcement (PSA) video on a health topic that is relevant to all professions. Peer review through an in-class presentation of these video projects has been essential to improving student engagement and quality of work. A key part of the video project is a team paper that outlines the peer-reviewed evidence in the video, cites the sources of the evidence, and explains how the team worked to develop the project.

IPE programs also can address the scale of introductory learning experiences by creating seminar courses that have multiple sections, each with a faculty facilitator. This can be an excellent method to increase student engagement and address difficult topics such as ethics or conflict management. A challenge of this type of learning experience is that it requires a great deal of faculty and administrative resources. Additionally, consistency in the pedagogy is a concern with multiple faculty members facilitating activities in different sections of the course.

Resource availability is a consistent theme in the IPE literature, and table 2.2 illustrates options for programs based on the level of institutional support. Faculty resources can be addressed through stipends or workload buyout by central administration. Another means of making faculty resources available is for the respective academic programs to provide faculty to serve on these teaching teams, building this time into their workload. This approach is effective if the programs

COLLABORATIVE CORNER
Opening Team Activity in an Introductory IPE Course

Write a brief bio for each team member:
- What do you most have in common?
- What unique attributes do you each bring to your team?

Respond to the following questions for your interprofessional team in this class:
- How will you communicate with each other?
- How will you evaluate whether your team is working well together?

Based on Eliot et al. (2018).

are committed to providing faculty resources that correlate to the number of students from their program in the IPE courses. Added value can be provided to these faculty members through collaborative research and scholarship opportunities, as well as by counting IPE teaching toward promotion and tenure requirements. Administrative resources most often are funded from an institutional commitment to the IPE program. These resources include administrative personnel time, priority room scheduling, and budgeted monies for supplies and technology. Pedagogical inconsistency is addressed through explicit development of teaching materials, faculty development, and regular teaching team meetings to coordinate content.

Advanced IPE Experiences (Late Learners, Kirkpatrick Levels 3-4)

Programs also incorporate advanced IPE courses to take what is learned in the introductory experiences and apply it in a more relevant context. These advanced experiences are not merely a reteaching of the concepts from the introductory course; rather, the instructional design requires that students operationalize their previous learning in an applicable setting.[30]

These courses can be developed specifically to serve this purpose or can exist as cross-listed or multidisciplinary courses in which parallel learning pedagogy is revised and repurposed with interprofessional design where learners from two or more professions learn about, from, and with each other. As a best practice, this approach calls for a teaching team with content expertise representing the mix of health professions using the course. However, MPE is commonly misconceived as IPE by educators just becoming acquainted with the concept. Simply blending classrooms (via cross-listed courses) of two professions does not ensure an effective IPE experience; the IPE plan must be deliberate, a framework of intentional skill-building activities that are measurable with a learning-level set of objectives achievable across the blended professions.[54]

There are many examples of higher-level IPE learning experiences:

• *Health care policy and system change*—Knowledge of health care systems and policy along with the fundamentals for advocacy and change agency can be presented to students learning in interprofessional teams. This course is designed to build on collaboration skills presented in an earlier introductory course. High-impact learning experiences in this type of course may include a poverty simulation or mock grant proposal for a program to improve health outcomes in an underserved community.

• *Quality improvement (QI) activities*—QI activities can be widely applied across health professions. They usually focus on improving an existing process or developing a new process to address a concern discovered through an evaluation process or an adverse event. This is an especially useful activity where learners from varied levels and contexts are brought together in an interprofessional learning experience. High-impact activities can include conducting interviews, debriefing, and making a group presentation to peers and other external stakeholders.[56]

• *Health care ethics and clinical decision making*—Clinical decision making and the bioethical concerns that inform those decisions can provide a rich learning environment for interprofessional teams. Core principles of health care, such as evidence-based practice, patient autonomy, and person-centered care, can be presented to diverse teams in this type of course. High-impact learning experiences include use of standardized patients, debate, guided reflection, and debriefing.[57]

• *Research and evidence-based practice*—Evidence-based practice provides the foundation for clinical practice in all health professions. Engaging in collaborative research, searching for best evidence, analyzing search results, and reporting findings can be effectively presented in an interprofessional course. Guided team-

EBP OF TEAMSHIP
Active IPE in a Patient-Based Setting

When considering teamwork in clinical training, real-life scenarios can be incredibly helpful in developing teamwork skills. In an example from Hallin and colleagues, students who participated in the practical application of teamwork in real-life patient care showed an increase in perceived improved knowledge of their own professional role as well as the roles of their interprofessional peers.[55] In a 2-week course, students participated in the care of patients both individually and as a team and were encouraged to develop processes for interprofessional team meetings, joint care planning, and team communication with the patient and family, all while relying on the other professions to assist in the care of the patient. When possible, faculty should consider opportunities for students to learn in teams in applied patient contexts.

based research on a relevant topic that applies to multiple professions provides a high-impact learning experience in this type of course.[58]

• *Medical humanities, communication, and health literacy*—The study of history, philosophy, theology, art, and literature can provide health professionals with a unique perspective on their work and their position in society. This approach can also be a useful way for health professionals to hear patients' and families' voices. It can be effective for learners at multiple levels: early learners, older students, or practicing clinicians. These activities also define the health care team more widely, beyond commonly accepted hierarchies and roles. High-impact activities can include debate, critical review, guided reflection, and debriefing.[59]

• *Grand rounds and case management*—Grand rounds are a traditional method where multiple health professionals come together to discuss cases and learn together. They can be applied in IPE with various levels of participation. Learners can watch grand rounds and reflect on the process, they can participate in a mock case or with standardized patients, or they can discuss an actual case they encounter in the clinical learning environment. High-impact activities include a root-cause analysis, where learners investigate and analyze actions by health professionals in an adverse event, and discussion of a case with complicated differential diagnoses or ethical considerations.[60]

Clinically Integrated IPE

Clinically integrated IPE is designed to directly improve the skills of IPCP through engagement in clinically relevant activities with learners from other programs. Participants appreciate the opportunity to authentically translate their profession-specific cognitive skills into clinical practice. Clinically integrated IPE manifests in many ways and is often correlated with resources, learner levels, and the mix of professional programs participating in the IPE plan. Activities such as clinical simulations, large-scale disaster simulations, simulated grand rounds, and case reviews are examples of clinically integrated IPE learning activities.[61,62] Clinical immersion activities such as community engagement, service learning, student-run clinics, and intentionally designed interprofessional clinics are also used to provide real experience with collaborative clinical practice.[63,64] Documentation of interprofessional collaboration in the participants' clinical practicum experiences is suggested to articulate the clinically integrated IPE.[65,66] High-impact clinical learning activities use portfolios to track and assess the activities. These portfolios can provide a student-centered method to track student progress and learning, especially when at clinical sites and participating remotely through other campuses.

However, there are many logistical challenges to the development and implementation of these activities.[67] One of the most important logistical challenges is constructing activities where the learning experience is consistent, reproducible, and assessable.[68] Programs have responded to this challenge by explicitly defining the tasks and expectations of students and faculty facilitators.[69] Facilitator training is also essential to the success of IPE clinical activities.[70-72] Programs looking for assistance with these training programs have many options. Examples of training programs include IPEC workshops, Train the Trainer (T3) courses, and TeamSTEPPS training.[72] See chapter 3 for more examples of IPE facilitator development.

Summary

IPE has numerous and varied models of delivery. Overall, IPE programs should be grounded in theory; provide opportunities for students to learn about, from, and with each other; and be formally assessed. Pedagogy designed to help learners from multiple professional programs learn about, from, and with each other requires intentional design to provide authentic collaborative learning. These learning activities, best cocreated by an interprofessional teaching team, must consider profession mix, learner level, institutional context, and available resources. They can occur in face-to-face, remote or online, or clinical settings. Reflection and debriefing are essential to optimizing the impact of these activities on student learning. Assessment is a necessary component of IPE and can provide opportunities for collaborative scholarship. It is hoped that IPE can help prepare collaboration-ready health professionals to enter a dynamic, evolving health care system.

Chapter 2 has provided a thorough grounding in the tenets of IPE and some of the models used in delivery. The next chapter presents professional development, examining the models, competencies, initiatives, and continuing professional education necessary for IPE and IPCP success.

CASE STUDY Debriefing

The faculty members of New City University soon realize they need a multilevel approach to IPE. Undergraduate learning experiences can be provided in a face-to-face, large-scale setting to accommodate large programs and varied learners. Graduate learning experiences can be designed as seminar courses, online courses, and clinically integrated learning experiences. Portfolio-based assessment may provide a valuable student-centered method to document and assess competencies and learning objectives. Institutional commitment to providing resources and faculty development is essential in the design of IPE activities. Faculty champions must be identified and supported as they collaborate to provide an effective and dynamic program of study that not only meets accreditation standards but also is transformative for graduates as they enter their respective health professions.

Case Study Discussion Questions

1. Buy-in from others is critical to the development and implementation of IPE curricula. What opportunities exist to create buy-in from the team?
2. With programs residing in different colleges, what factors need to be considered when designing the IPE program?
3. How does the availability of resources affect the implementation of IPE pedagogy?
4. What can be done to make IPE learning experiences more relevant for students from diverse programs?
5. How does the level of learner influence the choice of IPE pedagogy and mode of instruction?

CHAPTER 3

Interprofessional Development for Clinicians, Preceptors, and Faculty

Jordan Hamson-Utley, PhD, LAT, ATC

Objectives

After reading this chapter, the reader will be able to do the following:

- Illustrate the value of developing IPCP skills through IPE.
- Plan a pathway for professional development within IPE.
- Connect professional accreditation standards regarding IPE and IPCP to a culture of lifelong learning focused on teaming and collaborative practice in the workplace.
- Describe characteristics of faculty development programs designed to facilitate IPE.
- Gather recommendations for development, delivery, and assessment of IPE programs.

CASE STUDY Lifelong Learning

Joel has served 40 years as head athletic trainer at the high school in his hometown. Jan, a family nurse practitioner (FNP) who is the new nurse at his school, has accepted a student, Molly, from an FNP university program for a clinical rotation at the high school. Molly is in her final rotation and has completed all skills with high marks; she is also credentialed as an emergency medical technician (EMT). Shortly after Molly starts her rotation, she runs into Joel in the hallway and Jan makes the introductions. Joel is passive and disinterested in meeting Molly, as evidenced by his

(continued)

tone and body language, even after Jan requests his collaboration on an orthopedic case that occurred earlier that morning. Joel walks away, with little indication that he will follow up with them on the case. He fails to do so and avoids interactions with Jan, as usual.

Later that week, an emergency situation presents on the athletic field when a groundskeeper catches his hand in the blade of the lawn-mowing equipment, losing a few fingers. Joel responds quickly, activating the emergency response system through the high school police officer and then heading to the field. After several minutes Jan and Molly arrive at the field, where Joel is managing the situation by himself, collecting the amputated digits and instructing the groundskeeper to stay seated.

Following the incident, Joel, Jan, and Molly discuss the situation with the police officer as they write the incident report. Jan turns to Joel and says, "We could have helped you manage the situation, but we didn't want to step on your toes."

Learning how to work together as an effective team is essential to the delivery of health care. Like medicine itself, the delivery of care changes rapidly based on new laws, policies, and health care innovation. Staying level with change requires a pathway of development and a lifelong learning mind-set. Unfortunately, Joel is not an anomaly; a clinician who is stuck in the old ways of doing things often resists learning with, about, and from other members of the health care team. Luckily, Joel's reluctance to partner with Jan and Molly on previous cases had a limited impact on the care the groundskeeper received. However, there are many cases where the failure to work together well on patient care results in a devastating outcome.

Health care is a team sport. Just as sport requires athleticism and sport-specific skills operating in synergy toward a goal, health care teams require captains, diverse skill sets, and coordination to improve a patient's health. In basketball, could a team of only point guards beat a championship team? This might be the health care equivalent of a team of only PTs providing care for a patient after a stroke, for example. Additionally, IPCP is essential for health care teams to achieve patient care goals. Each position on a team requires a unique set of skills; without a point guard, a basketball team would lack leadership, ball vision, communication, and a 3-point scoring threat. Similarly, without a case lead, a care team would lack leadership, planning, communication, and an opportunity to win by providing the best patient care possible.

Graduating team-ready health care professionals requires seasoned educators, those who are experts in best practices not only in the classroom but also in IPE facilitation. As a result of limited experience in IPE facilitation, many educators are slowing the adoption of IPE[1] and potentially limiting the capacity of graduates to be ready to practice in a contemporary workplace. Literature to date is limited (but growing) in the area of faculty development for IPE, and existing research is not adequate to consider any method a best practice.[2] However, promising findings across existing methodologies indicate the value of modeling IPE knowledge, skills, and attitudes (KSAs); group work; reflection; and appreciation of diversity.[1]

Educator development is a critical component in the effective delivery of IPE. For an interprofessional team to achieve its purpose, it must capitalize on the diverse

COLLABORATIVE CORNER
Thoughtful Approach to IPE

When examining your pre- or postlicensure curriculum, it will become apparent that not all topics are suitable for IPE. There are certain roles that a single profession is tasked with executing in the clinical setting, and these topics should appear less often, if at all, in IPE curricula. Choose subject matter that calls for a team effort or relies on an interprofessional approach to provide patient care. Additionally, not every program or profession needs to be involved in every IPE opportunity. When programs are new to IPE, there is a tendency to be overly inclusive, gathering as many professions as possible for each opportunity on the premise that everyone will benefit. Be thoughtful in your approach to IPE to maximize its impact on learners and minimize organizational fatigue to sustain the effort.

knowledge and skills of the team. Delivering educator training in a collaborative framework affords exposure to teammates that promotes learning about each other, from each other, and with each other to devise strategies and solve problems related to classroom delivery or team-based patient care. The literature has established that continuing education that isolates health care professions prevents clinicians from developing collaborative capacities that meet the challenges of today's workplace.[3,4] Programs that deliver learning using a teaming approach are best positioned to benefit from the role models and networks that are built into this approach. Faculty and clinicians who are expected to engage in IPE and the team-based learning of future clinicians must be supported with the knowledge and skills necessary to design and facilitate IPE.[5]

Faculty KSAs and Behavioral Change

IPE educator development programs aim to improve KSAs (knowledge, skills, and attitudes), as well as influence resulting behaviors by health care graduates in the workplace. Improving KSAs is a standard goal of professional development in IPE[6-10] (see chapter 2 for a list of IPEC core competencies). Research assessing attitudes and skills is considered level 2 evidence, and translation to patient care cannot be assumed. As indicated by Kirkpatrick's levels of outcomes[11] for IPE programs, changes in participant (level 3) and organizational (level 4a) behavior anchor the top half of the pyramid and correlate with creating positive change in health care delivery. Figure 3.1 illustrates the levels of assessment applied to IPE. Few professional development programs assess changes at the behavior level (center of the pyramid and above). Those that meet the challenge examine roles and responsibilities,[12] interprofessional communication,[13] and teamwork.[12] The majority of research to date has assessed reactions and changes in attitudes and perceived knowledge; however, the translation of knowledge to behavioral change and resulting improvements in patient care is the ultimate goal of IPE.[10,14,15]

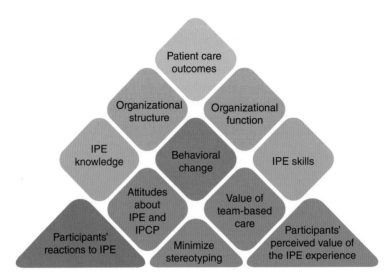

Figure 3.1   Kirkpatrick's levels of assessment applied to IPE.

EBP OF TEAMSHIP
Moving IPE Forward

Findings from a 2018 systematic review of the nursing literature indicated that a surge in IPE research is apparent, albeit the designs are weak, resulting in minimal influence on the interprofessional development of health care clinicians.[2] Adding to the problem, the various tools used to assess IPE effectiveness lack repetition across studies, making it more difficult to compare results across populations. Clouding the waters a bit more, a lack of appropriate psychometrics, or no evidence of validation beyond the initial study, was also apparent in this review; using tools that are not effective in assessing IPE leaves uninterruptable and ungeneralizable results. Potentially slowing the IPE movement the most, the level of assessment (Kirkpatrick's levels 1-4) in this review found all studies reported level 1 (reactions to IPE) and level 2 (IPE attitudes and knowledge) assessments, while no studies reported level 3 or 4 assessments. IPE research that documents behavioral change (level 3) or reports transfer of knowledge that influences patient care outcomes (level 4) is both critical and compulsory to move IPE forward.

Knowledge and Skills as Barriers

As mentioned earlier, lack of knowledge about IPE can pose a barrier to implementation; additionally, educators may not have the skills to facilitate IPE.[16] Positive changes in attitudes are often reported alongside increased knowledge of peer professions in health care. Professional development and formal IPE afford opportunities to increase the knowledge and skills necessary to participate in and lead or facilitate interprofessional teams. Consider another example involving PT and OT programs within the same university using multiprofessional education (MPE) instead of IPE. One profession is willing to engage in IPE while the other wishes to separate the MPE classroom experiences to gain better control over the learning experiences. It can be assumed that the profession wishing to disengage from MPE lacks respect for the peer profession, discounting the value of intermixing the students from both professions. Who loses in this case?

Valuing diversity in an interprofessional faculty is an important competency in IPE delivery.[16] Allowing time for health care peers to get to know each other builds capacity and sustainability for IPE.[18] During educator workshops, it is important to highlight that when delivering IPE, facilitation skills become paramount and should be emphasized beyond skills of an individual profession.[19] Furthermore, evidence suggests networking with health care peers during professional development sessions is highly valuable.[20] Learners must understand their role and the roles of their teammates during IPE preparation; the intention of educating professionals in a team framework is that these identified roles will transfer to work in collaborative teams (in the classroom or in the clinic). For example, athletic training is often confused with personal training or weightlifting (which may be offensive to athletic trainers, who are experts in orthopedic evaluation). A simple conversation in a nonthreatening environment clears up this ambiguity and builds the foundation for respect and trust.

Additionally, if faculty members are confused about each other's qualifications or roles, it will likely affect their students. As a result, networking is commonly found in effective IPE professional development models,[1] and the relationships (and attitudes and knowledge) built should be modeled for students.

COLLABORATIVE CORNER
Why Do We Use MPE?

MPE refers to blending students from two or more professions in a single classroom to learn alongside one another, in parallel, without planned interaction.[17] There is likely only one reason this occurs in higher education and in clinical settings: Paying one educator to meet the needs of students from multiple programs checks the financial responsibility box. However, might this always be a missed opportunity? Consider topics that are taught in higher education to students from multiple academic programs, such as accounting, finance, anatomy, and pathophysiology. What is stopping the educator from connecting the dots between the future professionals in the course? Is there no perceived value in an aspiring accountant learning from an entrepreneur, or a nursing student learning from a dental hygienist in training? When is it too early to expose students to real-life collaboration? The value proposition is not likely the deterrent; it's more likely educator development (individual) and resulting learning objectives (organizational) that force the instructor to connect the dots.

TOOLS OF IPE
Team Huddle

Team-building exercises are a common component of IPE educator development programs. They promote knowledge exchange by team members, usually geared toward solving problems in a collaborative fashion. The interactions aim to reduce misconceptions and stereotypes about fellow health care professionals. A team huddle[21] can be used at the beginning of a training program as an icebreaker or as a way to promote discussion at a lunch between sessions. To use this exercise, first form interprofessional teams. Then, task the teams with solving a complex patient care case while promoting IPCP, reducing cost, and optimizing care. All members must respond to the case through a team-huddle discussion. Their responses must include their profession's role in the case, their readiness or experience as a profession to collaborate on team care, and any personal or professional strengths they bring to the case. Following the huddle, teams present their patient care plan to the large group. To enrich professional development opportunities, the team huddle can be paired with knowledge dissemination on education and certification or licensure for each health care profession.

Attitudes as a Barrier

Although strides are being made toward widespread implementation of IPE across professional health care curricula, academic elitism remains,[5] posing a threat to effective execution of IPE. The notion that one health profession is more important or performs more valuable skills than another limits inclusion and team performance, ultimately inhibiting patient care and safety. To gain context, consider the health care fields of athletic training and physical therapy, highly complementary in the rehabilitation of patients. Some professional curricula use MPE or IPE with cofacilitation and share clinical sites for student rotations, whereas other programs stay separate, even in the face of accreditation mandates that require interprofessional exposure. Ego, elitism, and negative attitudes toward peer professions in health care limit the impact that programs and educators can have on the next generation of change agents in health care.

Attitudes of health care providers toward IPE are arguably the best predictor of intent to engage in collaborative education and practice.[22] Research shows that most health care educators hold positive attitudes toward IPE,[22-24,77] and those attitudes can be changed through education,[20,25] including online education.[26] Additionally, gender and age may influence attitudes of interprofessional team members. Research has revealed that women hold more positive attitudes toward IPE[23,27] compared with their male counterparts; however, not all research examining gender differences has found significant results.[22]

TOOLS OF IPE
Modified Readiness for Interprofessional Learning Scale (mRIPLS)

This tool is used to assess clinicians' attitudes toward IPE and to determine the effectiveness of a learning experience. The original version of this tool, the Readiness for Interprofessional Learning Scale (RIPLS), was created for use with health professional students.[29] It was modified for use with post-certification professionals to assess their beliefs toward IPE and IPCP.[30] The mRIPLS consists of 23 statements scored on a 5-point Likert scale by summing 3 subscales: teamwork and collaboration (TWC), patient-centeredness (PC), and sense of professional identity (PI). Use with practicing athletic trainers yielded internal consistency of the mRIPLS as acceptable (alpha = 0.872); internal consistency of each subscale resulted in TWC (alpha = 0.917), PC (alpha = 0.862), and PI (alpha = 0.632), of which the PI subscale was reported to be unacceptable.[30]

Regarding age, the literature is split on the effect of age on attitudes toward IPE[22,23]; however, intuition suggests that as health care practitioners gain experience and expertise, they will be exposed to interprofessional team care and see the value in collaboration. Implications exist, then, for young professionals without extensive experience or expertise; newly licensed clinicians may not have positive attitudes toward IPE, predicting their intent to engage.[22] However, new clinicians graduating from academic programs with a strong IPE curriculum are likely to have positive KSAs regarding IPE. Additionally, faculty members who seek IPE facilitator development show significantly improved KSAs.[18-20,25,28] A starting point for programs seeking to develop facilitators is to assess readiness to engage in IPE by sampling current attitudes toward and perceptions about the value of IPE. Implementing educational interventions aimed at addressing common misconceptions and building bridges between health care professions are a likely next step.

Development Models and Interprofessional Competencies

Without a defined best practice for IPE, those active in IPE facilitator development turn to WHO (World Health Organization),[31] IPEC (Interprofessional Education Collaborative),[14] and NAM (National Academy of Medicine),[32] as well as the professional standards for prelicensure requirements of students in their specific health care field,[33-40] to guide their personal development. This makes intuitive sense; if they are to facilitate the learning of team-based care, for example, they must achieve advanced learning in effective teams, collaboration, team leadership, and team-based care. The Professional Education Standards Related to IPE sidebar presents standards for quick reference to the language used to describe IPE and IPCP, and in some cases it illustrates special requirements for students entering advanced levels of their profession (e.g., nursing). It is through these standards that health care professions will align into efficient patient care teams. As evidenced in the sidebar, some professions have more work to do than others (e.g., athletic training, PA) to prepare their graduates to be effective members of an interprofessional team; this may also be true of the development of faculty and educators in those professions. Development of IPE initiatives must also consider the involvement and training of staff, faculty, and administration, as well as implementation logistics such as curricular content, scheduling, and cross-program learning objectives.

PROFESSIONAL EDUCATION STANDARDS RELATED TO IPE

Athletic Training[33]

- *Standard 8*—Planned IPE is incorporated within the professional program.
- *Standard 61*—Practice in collaboration with other health care and wellness professionals.

Dietetics[34]

- *KRDN 2.2*—Describe the governance of nutrition and dietetics practice, such as the scope of nutrition and dietetics practice and the code of ethics for the profession of nutrition and dietetics, and describe interprofessional relationships in various practice settings.
- *KRDN 2.5*—Identify and describe the work of interprofessional teams and the roles of others with whom the registered dietitian or nutritionist collaborates in the delivery of food and nutrition services.
- *CRDN 2.4*—Function as a member of interprofessional teams.

Nursing[35]

- *Doctor of Nursing Practice (DNP) Essential VI*—Interprofessional collaboration for improving patient and population health outcomes. Today's complex health care environment depends on the contributions of highly skilled and knowledgeable individuals from multiple professions. In order to accomplish the IOM mandate for safe, timely, effective, efficient, equitable, and patient-centered care in a complex environment, health care professionals must function as highly collaborative teams.
- *Master of Science in Nursing (MSN) Essential VII*—Interprofessional collaboration for improving patient and population health outcomes. The MSN communicates, collaborates, and consults with other health professionals to manage and coordinate care.

Occupational Therapy (OT)[36]

Doctor of Occupational Therapy (OTD)

- Be prepared to effectively communicate and work interprofessionally with those who provide care for individuals or populations in order to clarify each member's responsibility in executing components of an intervention plan.

- Effectively communicate, coordinate, and work interprofessionally with those who provide services to individuals, organizations, or populations in order to clarify each member's responsibility in executing components of an intervention plan.

Master of Occupational Therapy (MOT)

- Be prepared to effectively communicate and work interprofessionally with those who provide care for individuals or populations in order to clarify each member's responsibility in executing components of an intervention plan.

- Effectively communicate and work interprofessionally with those who provide services to individuals, organizations, or populations in order to clarify each member's responsibility in executing an intervention plan.

Pharmacology[37]

- *Standard 3.4: Interprofessional collaboration*—The graduate is able to actively participate and engage as a health care team member by demonstrating mutual respect, understanding, and values to meet patient care needs.

- *Standard 11.1: Interprofessional team dynamics*—All students demonstrate competence in interprofessional team dynamics, including articulating the values and ethics that underpin interprofessional practice; engaging in effective interprofessional communication, including conflict resolution and documentation skills; and honoring interprofessional roles and responsibilities. Interprofessional team dynamics are introduced, reinforced, and practiced in the didactic and Introductory Pharmacy Practice Experience (IPPE) components of the curriculum, and competency is demonstrated in Advanced Pharmacy Practice Experience (APPE) practice settings.

- *Standard 11.2: Interprofessional team education*—To advance collaboration and quality of patient care, the didactic and experiential curricula include opportunities for students to learn about, from, and with other members of the interprofessional health care team. Through IPE activities, students gain an understanding of the abilities, competencies, and scope of practice of team members. Some, but not all, of these educational activities may be simulations.

(continued)

- *Standard 11.3: Interprofessional team practice*—All students competently participate as a health care team member in providing direct patient care and engaging in shared therapeutic decision making. They participate in experiential educational activities with prescribers and student prescribers and other student and professional health care team members, including face-to-face interactions that are designed to advance interprofessional team effectiveness.

- *Standard 12.5: IPPE expectations*—IPPEs expose students to common contemporary U.S. practice models, including interprofessional practice involving shared patient care decision making, professional ethics and expected behaviors, and direct patient care activities. IPPEs are structured and sequenced to intentionally develop a clear understanding of what constitutes exemplary pharmacy practice in the United States prior to beginning APPE.

- *Standard 12.6: IPPE duration*—IPPE totals no less than 300 clock hours of experience and is purposely integrated into the didactic curriculum. A minimum of 150 hours of IPPE are balanced between community and institutional health-system settings.

- *Standard 12.7: Simulation for IPPE*—Simulated practice experiences (a maximum of 60 clock hours of the total 300 hours) may be used to mimic actual or realistic pharmacist-delivered patient care situations. However, simulation hours do not substitute for the 150 clock hours of required IPPE time in community and institutional health-system settings. Didactic instruction associated with the implementation of simulated practice experiences is not counted toward any portion of the 300-hour IPPE requirement.

- *Standard 13.3: Interprofessional experiences*—In the aggregate, students gain in-depth experience in delivering direct patient care as part of an interprofessional team.

- *Standard 18.1: Sufficient faculty*—The college or school has a sufficient number of faculty members to effectively address the need for intraprofessional and interprofessional collaboration.

- *Standard 21.2: Physical facility attributes*—The college or school's physical facilities also include adequate pace that facilitates interaction of administrators, faculty, students, and interprofessional collaborators.

- *Standard 24.3: Student achievement and readiness*—The assessment plan measures student achievement at defined levels of the professional competencies that support attainment of the educational outcomes in aggregate and at the individual student level. In addition to college- or school-desired assessments, the plan includes an assessment of student readiness to contribute as a member of an interprofessional collaborative patient care team.

- *Standard 25.6: Interprofessional preparedness*—The college or school assesses the preparedness of all students to function effectively and professionally on an interprofessional health care team.

- *Interprofessional interaction*—The need for interprofessional interaction is paramount to successful treatment of patients. Colleges and schools provide pharmacy students the opportunity to gain interprofessional skills using a variety of mechanisms, including face-to-face interactions in clinical settings or in real-time telephonic or video-linked interactions. Regardless of the methods used, students demonstrate those interprofessional skills articulated in Standard 11.

Physical Therapy (PT)[38]

- *Standard 6F*—The didactic and clinical curriculum includes IPE; learning activities are directed toward the development of interprofessional competencies including, but not limited to, values and ethics, communication, professional roles and responsibilities, and teamwork.
  - Describe learning activities that involve students, faculty, or practitioners from other health care professions.
  - Describe the effectiveness of the learning activities in preparing students and graduates for team-based collaborative care.

- *Standard 6L*—The curriculum plan includes clinical education experiences for each student that encompass, but are not limited to, the following:
  - *6L3*—Involvement in interprofessional practice
    - Describe the program's expectation for opportunities for involvement in interprofessional practice during clinical experiences.
    - Provide evidence that students have opportunities for interprofessional practice.

- *Standard 7D*—The physical therapist professional curriculum includes content and learning experiences designed to prepare students to achieve educational outcomes required for initial practice

(continued)

of physical therapy. Courses within the curriculum include content designed to prepare program students to do the following:

- *7D7*—Communicate effectively with all stakeholders, including patients and clients, family members, caregivers, practitioners, interprofessional team members, consumers, payers, and policymakers.
- *7D28*—Manage the delivery of the plan of care that is consistent with professional obligations, interprofessional collaborations, and administrative policies and procedures of the practice environment.
- *7D37*—Assess and document safety risks of patients and the health care provider and design and implement strategies to improve safety in the health care setting as an individual and as a member of the interprofessional health care team.
- *7D39*—Participate in patient-centered IPCP.

Physician Assistant (PA)[39]

- *B1.08*—The curriculum *must* include instruction to prepare students to work collaboratively in interprofessional patient-centered teams.

Speech Language Pathology (SLP)[40]

3.1.1B Professional Practice Competencies

The program must provide content and opportunities for students to learn so that each student can demonstrate the following attributes and abilities and demonstrate those attributes and abilities in the manners identified.

Accountability

- Understand how to work on interprofessional teams to maintain a climate of mutual respect and shared values.

Effective Communication

- Communicate—with patients, families, communities, interprofessional team colleagues, and other professionals caring for individuals—in a responsive and responsible manner that supports a team approach to maximize care outcomes.

Professional Duty

- Understand the roles and importance of interdisciplinary or interprofessional assessment and intervention and be able to interact and coordinate care effectively with other disciplines and community resources.

Collaborative Practice
- Understand how to apply values and principles of interprofessional team dynamics.
- Understand how to perform effectively in different interprofessional team roles to plan and deliver care—centered on the individual served—that is safe, timely, efficient, effective, and equitable.

3.1.4A Assessment of the Structure and Function of the Auditory and Vestibular Systems

The program provides academic content and clinical education experiences so that each student can learn and demonstrate knowledge and skills in order to engage in interprofessional practice to facilitate optimal assessment of the individual being served.

3.1.6A Intervention to Minimize the Effects of Changes in the Auditory and Vestibular Systems on an Individual's Ability to Participate in the Environment

The curriculum provides academic content and clinical education experiences so that each student can learn and demonstrate knowledge and skills in order to conduct audiologic (re)habilitation and engage in interprofessional practice to maximize outcomes for individuals served.

Core Principles of IPE Professional Development

The Josiah Macy Jr. Foundation guides the efforts of organizations to develop IPE facilitators through the following broad recommendation: "Expand faculty development programs to prepare health professionals for effective interprofessional learning, teaching, and practice."[41(p29)] A more descriptive approach from IPEC includes the core competencies for IPCP (noted in chapter 2).[14] IPEC outlined its faculty development initiatives to include 10 institutes hosted since 2012; these institutes focused on advancing IPE at the participant's setting (e.g., workplace, clinic, hospital, university) and hosted 339 teams (1,457 participants) from 185 cities, 48 states, and 4 countries (including the United States, Lebanon, South Africa, and Canada). The 2016 update revised the 2011 framework following work by Englander and colleagues, who defined a common set of competencies for physicians, shaping the existing 4 core competencies (and corresponding subcompetencies; see chapter 2) under a single domain, the Interprofessional Collaborative Domain.[14(p10)] Many professional development programs target a single competency,[20,25,42,43] while others take a more comprehensive approach to develop all of the competencies.[18,19,28,44,45] When designing IPE faculty development, the topic and depth of the dive determine the options for delivery.

Delivery Models

While professional education makes strides to stay current with the demands of the rapidly changing health care landscape, faculty development models for IPE and practice are scarce.[46] IPEC has called for an increase in faculty development initiatives to help educators facilitate the development of collaboration-ready clinicians.[14] Delivery methods include both face-to-face and online models with various interactive pedagogies such as role-play,[47,28] case-based learning,[47-51] and grand rounds.[52] Related, facilitator development initiatives should aim to promote change at both the individual and organizational levels[5]; however, the secret sauce that drives effective IPCP is the team.

Interprofessional Group Dynamics

Managing a landscape of diverse groups requires effective IPE facilitation, especially in educator development sessions. Encouraging a heterogeneous group of health care professionals to work collaboratively toward a shared goal is challenging; however, when groups fail to collaborate, it negatively affects job satisfaction, patient outcomes, and resource use.[53] Understanding that the learners' knowledge and experience will affect how they function in a group is fundamental for an IPE facilitator. Designing interprofessional teams for workshop collaborations requires consideration beyond just the health care profession of the learner. Years of professional health care experience (often correlated with age) may also affect the IPE experience. Consider this: How often in the workplace does a health care team have all new graduates on the roster? If it does, what might the team members struggle with or what mistakes might they make? On the other hand, how might years of experience play into the efficiency of a care team? What about gender or

EBP OF TEAMSHIP
Cofacilitation in the Classroom

The benefits of collaborating on teams are seen not only in patient care but also in the classroom as well.[54] Research on faculty development suggests that educators who lead IPE are better facilitators if they have experience working on teams[55]; they respect and value individual differences, they are self-aware, and they are conscious of group dynamics and their impact on learning. Additionally, using a pair of facilitators, or cofacilitation, is a common strategy in IPE.[55] Receiving instruction from a smooth-operating dyad, a pair that complements each other's styles and facilitates effectively, models best-practice teamship in the classroom. This type of modeling is often missing in the student's clinical setting and has been called a critical factor in the success of IPE.

ethnicity? All of these factors influence team dynamics and should be considered when designing IPE workshop teams that parallel real-life teams with the purpose of maximizing learner impact. To explain further, professional experience allows teammates to learn from each other's mistakes and successes and promotes the notion of group knowledge through collaboration.

Coaching diverse learners to be open-minded and stay focused on the proposed outcomes of the IPE session may afford increases in KSAs toward IPE[56]; hence, the importance of developing skills in IPE facilitation. The facilitator must be an effective leader and have a positive attitude, expect positive change, create a safe and trusting environment, and facilitate positive relations between professions to achieve the positive results of group work (i.e., improved teaming).[44] A final point to consider regarding the impact of training in groups: With effective facilitation, small interprofessional group learning activities offer interactions that simulate real-life teamwork.

Power of Reflection

IPE educator development models that afford time for self- and peer-reflection have led to increased KSAs related to IPE.[5,16,18,55,56] In addition, reflection is an essential ingredient for improving KSAs related to facilitation of IPE.[16,46,55,57] Educators are busy people; building in time for reflection in a 3-day retreat or creating a formal review session after a series of 1-hour lunch-and-learn sessions is essential to improve knowledge and skill translation into classroom facilitation. For example, opportunities to share across professions (and classrooms) what did and didn't work have the potential to strengthen the IPE initiative and move it forward at a faster pace.

EBP OF TEAMSHIP
The Evidence: Student and Faculty Reflection

"I appreciated the emphasis on IPE and participation in problem-solving with students from various backgrounds. I very much enjoyed all of the course assignments and activities as they were relevant to real-world experiences, facilitated peer interaction and problem solving, and emphasized interprofessional practice." —IPE student, course evaluation, fall 2018

"I bring over 20 years of health care experience into the classroom. As a nurse, I have experience collaborating on care teams and know the value of this to the [health care] system and the patient. It is essential for both pre- and postlicense students to be exposed to developing their professional skills and their team skills; balancing the two, finding time to develop both is challenging for faculty." —IPE course contributing faculty Dr. Stefi Podlog, spring 2019

Organizational Models and Initiatives

To be sustainable, IPE initiatives should be tethered to a strategic plan or interwoven into the language of the university's mission. Additionally, gleaning support from department or university-level administrators seems to be a key to success.[46] IPE is a philosophy; it is a method of delivering health professions education that goes beyond meeting standards and essentials for the accreditor. One piece of evidence that an academic organization has fully embraced IPE as central to its mission is when IPE facilitation and curriculum development are reflected in promotion and tenure guidelines[46]; this is consistent with suggestions made by the Josiah Macy Jr. Foundation in a postconference summary report. The foundation made the following recommendations for professional development[41(pp28-29)]:

- Reform the education and lifelong career development of health professionals to incorporate interprofessional learning and team-based care.
- Expand faculty development programs to prepare health professionals for effective interprofessional learning, teaching, and practice.
- Incorporate interprofessional team-based competencies in performance reviews of health professionals in clinical and academic settings.

Furthermore, creating a network of IPE facilitators through professional development is essential to sustaining the momentum following annual offerings. What follows is a series of examples of professional development models aimed at increasing the KSAs of IPE facilitators.

The professional development models showcased in this chapter are examples for organizations (e.g., universities, hospitals) to prepare and position facilitators to make an impact on IPE and clinical practice. Future research examining the effectiveness of such models is warranted to cultivate best practice recommendations for faculty development. Somewhat promising, research summarized to date on student KSAs found a positive effect of IPE interventions across health care professions.[59] Faculty must now move to strengthen this finding across health care professions education to improve the readiness of graduates to collaborate on care teams.

Essentials Program

The Essentials program, a retreat-based immersion followed by a series of sessions offered by the Cleveland Clinic, was adapted from a generic educator development program and designed for delivery at an academic health care center.[58] The goals of the IPE development program are to enhance educators' skills and to create a local community of support for IPE facilitation (i.e., create a network). The program is based on adult learning theory and uses reflective practice, group work (with interprofessional peers), and experiential learning. The immersive element includes a 3-hour retreat kickoff on educational theory, followed by 25 bimonthly workshops (1.5-3 hours in length). Workshop topics include the following:

- Teaching skills
- Clinical reasoning

- Objective writing
- Curriculum design
- Effective feedback
- Competency-based education (CBE) and assessment
- Technology-based education

The program is open to all faculty and clinical instructors who teach prelicensed physicians, nurses, PAs, nutritionists, audiologists, perfusionists, and medical researchers. The program began in 2013 with 54 individuals and increased to 152 participants in 2016. Highest annual participation in this model was 570 total participants (in 2016), with a range of 6 to 41 per workshop. Workshops were assessed using a 10-item survey measuring workshop teaching techniques and personal learning on a 4-point Likert scale. Over 3 offering cycles, 944 surveys were collected from 1,134 total participants (83.4% response rate). Grand means

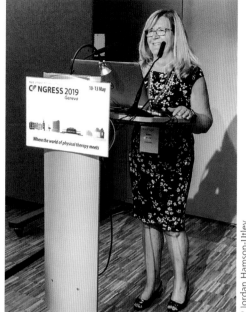

© Jordan Hamson-Utley

Dr. Karen Snyder, PhD, OTR/L, presents research findings on IPE at the 2019 World Confederation for Physical Therapy (WCPT) in Geneva, Switzerland.

from participants regarding workshop teaching techniques 3.5 to 4.0 ($M = 3.8$) and personal learning 3.35 to 4.0 ($M = 3.7$) were reported to align with a high degree of satisfaction with the program. No longitudinal follow-ups were mentioned.

Interprofessional Institute

The Interprofessional Institute model from the Medical University of South Carolina[46] may be the most common professional development model, where a theme is selected and then talks and activities are generated around the theme and delivered in sequence to faculty, adjunct faculty, and clinical preceptors. The model intentionally influences 3 key areas:

1. IPE education
2. IPE research
3. IPE practice

The institute is open to all interested educators from across 6 campuses, and 6 sessions are offered once a year:

1. Introduction to IPE
2. Value of interprofessional teams and team skills
3. Communication skills

4. Conflict resolution

5. Negotiation skills

6. Leading change

Participants take turns acting as facilitators at one of the sessions, which are 2.5 hours long (1.5 hours didactic with active learning, 1.0 hour reflection and project work). Also, participants are tasked with completing an interprofessional project and shadowing or interviewing someone from another health care profession. The evaluation of this model included a simple pre- and posttest IPE survey that found no significant differences in any of the subscales following completion of the institute. A longitudinal follow-up survey delivered 1 to 2 years later ($n = 36$) found that 69% of participants indicated increased involvement in interprofessional initiatives (80%, $n = 20$), interprofessional collaborations (64%, $n = 16$), and interprofessional scholarly activity (60%, $n = 15$). Participants ($n = 88$) identified with research ($n = 18$), clinical ($n = 25$), and education ($n = 45$) as their primary responsibility.[46]

Interprofessional Fellowship

Also developed by the Medical University of South Carolina, the Interprofessional Fellowship model[46] affords a deep dive into IPE collaboration, facilitation, and application and is intended for faculty who will lead interprofessional work in their department (e.g., teaching, research, administration). Two fellows are selected annually for the program through competitive application and are awarded a $5,000 stipend. Fellows participate in the Interprofessional Institute as facilitators and attend monthly group IPE mentoring sessions held across the academic year. The evaluation of this model was yet to be realized at the time of this writing. The fellows developed a new interprofessional course elective and completed an interprofessional project that was submitted for a grant.[46]

IPE Teaching Series

The IPE Teaching Series from the Medical University of South Carolina[46] focuses on improving teaching and facilitation skills in the IPE classroom. Participants are paired with a monthlong mentor who guides exploration of IPE and provides feedback on implementation strategies and assessment methods. Participants are offered 4 sessions:

1. IPEC competencies and instructional methods

2. IPE instructional design principles

3. IPE group facilitation

4. IPE evaluation and assessment methods

Each session lasts 1.5 hours (45 minutes didactic, 45 minutes application). Across the sessions, the participants work in teams to complete an interprofessional project. Evaluation of this model included survey data collection 1 month after the series concluded. The survey found more than 80% of participants ($n = 11$; 50% response rate) agreed that "as a result of the Interprofessional Teaching Series, I applied" national IPE competencies, delivery methods of IPE, instructional design for IPE, group facilitation skills for IPE, and assessment and evaluation methods for IPE.[46]

Train the Trainer (T3): Interprofessional Team Development Program

The T3 Interprofessional Team Development Program develops collaborative teams to transform health care education and practice with an in-person experiential education program followed by a year of consulting. Participants attend a 3.5-day session at 1 of the 3 national sites, followed by a series of online webinars and on-demand coaching calls. The longitudinal design of the program affords support beginning with the immersive session through the implementation of IPE and IPCP projects. The program is for educators, researchers, practitioners, students, and others who have an interest in bridging the research and training gaps between IPE and IPCP. This program was established with support from a grant from the Josiah Macy Jr. Foundation in collaboration with NCIPE. Following are the T3 learning objectives:

- Examine how interprofessional learning plays a role across the IOM learning continuum from classrooms to practice.
- Explore and practice skills that can help align interprofessional research and training in both education and practice settings.
- Network with interprofessional leaders to discuss lessons learned from coordinating interprofessional research and training across the learning continuum.

Assessing Continuing Professional Education

Assessing the effectiveness of IPE facilitator development is essential to inform best practice. As indicated in various systematic reviews of the effectiveness of IPE,[2,60,61] the lack of solid evidence is likely the result of weakness and heterogeneity of research design and the numerous assessment tools (some validated, some not) that exist today.

Tool repositories exist to guide IPE program administrators on assessment strategies by showcasing validated tools to collect data (i.e., KSAs, behaviors). One such site is the NCIPE, which can be located by using the following search term online: "Nexus IPE Resource Center". The Nexus was developed as an international information hub to support IPE and IPCP efforts. The site includes open-source access to validated tools for use in assessment of IPE and provides corresponding published manuscripts to support use in various settings.

Kirkpatrick's Expanded Outcomes Typology

In program evaluation, it is important to understand the type of change resulting from the IPE development program. Kirkpatrick's adapted evaluation model[56] outlines 4 levels of assessment; the higher the level, the more salient or authentic the assessment (table 3.1; see also figure 3.1).

- *Level 1*—The lowest level of the model assesses IPE through the reactions of participants. Assessments that gather only participants' reactions to IPE would be considered weak.
- *Level 2*—This level assesses the effectiveness of IPE by measuring changes in attitudes and perceptions (2a) as well as knowledge and skills (2b) related to IPE, IPCP, and teamwork. If participants hold a negative attitude, they may behave in a way that poses a barrier to effective teaming, limiting the potential of their team.
- *Level 3*—This level of assessment measures changes in participant behavior. This can be observed or self-reported behavioral change collected qualitatively or quantitatively.
- *Level 4*—This level of assessment measures change in organizational practice (4a) and outcomes related to both patients and learners (4b).

Most research to date has studied participants' reactions (level 1), attitude and perception changes (2a), and knowledge and skill gains (2b); this is the low-hanging fruit of IPE assessment.

Measuring reactions can be as simple as an online course evaluation. Attitude change can be examined using a pretest–posttest or retrospective pretest–posttest survey design. Potential limitations of assessment with surveys include self-reporting and various types of bias. However, assessment of knowledge and skill gains can take an objective approach using multiple-choice quizzes that measure competence with theory and definitions. Knowledge can also be assessed in combination with

Table 3.1 Kirkpatrick's Levels of Assessment Applied to IPE

Level	Measure	Related Outcomes
1	Reaction to IPE	Participants' perceptions of the IPE experience; value of the IPE experience
2a	Attitudes and perceptions related to IPE	IPE attitude changes or altered perceptions of other health care groups; attitudes about the value of team care
2b	Knowledge and skills related to IPE	Knowledge and skills that promote IPCP
3	Behavioral change related to IPE	Learning transfer to health care behaviors; influence on professional practice
4a	Change in organizational approach to IPE	Changes in organizational approach to patient care; structure and function
4b	Improvements in patient care, wellness outcomes	Improvements in health and well-being of patients being treated by interprofessional care teams

attitudes on survey tools. Programs should look to promote change in behaviors at the individual (3) and organizational (4a) levels, as well as improve the process of health care for the team and the patient (4b). Elements at levels 3 and 4 are more difficult to assess because they relate to behaviors; some IPCP and IPE questionnaires assess behavioral change from both individual and team vantage points (e.g., PACT [level 3],[62,63] ICAR [level 3],[27,64] ICCAS [level 3],[65] IPEC Competency Survey Instrument [level 3],[66] IIC [level 4a][67]). A 2017 systematic review of assessment tools for IPE reported that the highest level of assessment occurring in IPE professional development to date is level 4a.[60] See chapter 4 for a comprehensive list of assessment tools for IPE and IPCP.

TOOLS OF IPE
Interprofessional Collaborator Assessment Rubric (ICAR)

This tool is intended for use in the assessment of IPCP. Broadly, it assesses the following collaboration competencies:

- Communication
- Collaboration
- Roles and responsibilities
- Collaborative patient care
- Team functioning
- Conflict management and resolution

The development of ICAR was guided by an interprofessional advisory committee composed of educators from medicine, rehabilitative sciences, and nursing to be used across health care professions, at any level of education, as formative or summative assessment.[68]

A rubric benefits both the evaluator and the learner because levels of competency are clearly outlined. The tool should be used across multiple observation exposures, and users should create a remediation plan for learners who do not meet an acceptable level of competency.

The rubric was validated using typological analysis of interprofessional competency frameworks (national and international), a Delphi survey of IPE experts, and focus groups of students and educators. Use of ICAR to assess the impact of simulation learning on collaboration of medical students in Iran found an overall internal consistency of .71 (measured by computing Cronbach's alphas), and it found the individual subscales to range from .65 to .75, with a test–retest reliability of .76 overall, and the individual subscales to range from .73 to .83.[69] The rubric is 19 items and is open source, available online.

IPE Faculty Development as Lifelong Learning

For the sake of clarity, the term *faculty* will be used throughout this chapter to refer to those who teach in both clinical and university settings, in formal and informal ways, in classrooms or on teams. An essential ingredient of effective teaching is the consideration of best practices, which arise from research and examining the available literature. In this chapter, faculty development is presented in a way that can be applied across settings and professions, focusing on the assessment and development of KSAs regarding IPE.

A good starting point for devising a personal pathway of development is to examine the ideal characteristics of interprofessional educators. These include experience in group facilitation, team teaching, conflict resolution, and connection of theory to practice, on top of expertise in clinical practice.[56] In addition, being positive and enthusiastic, tech savvy, pragmatic, and a skilled communicator align with the talents of an effective educator. Educators must also be able to create authentic assessments and provide sensitive feedback, as well as implement data-driven change in the curriculum. Accrediting bodies have begun to mandate the inclusion of IPE in the prelicensure education of various health care professions.[70] As the accreditation initiative progresses across all health professions, educators must look for ways to become efficient in facilitating IPE. Similar to faculty, clinicians collaborating on teams may also need to seek out training on effective teaming.

Newly licensed clinicians who are operating in interprofessional frameworks were likely educated under standards that included interprofessional teaming, collaborative decision making, respect, trust, and use of common language in communication; moreover, leadership of interprofessional teams is a nursing essential and aligns with the postprofessional education of the MSN. It is fair to say that clinicians who entered their field prior to the appearance of IPCP in professional standards have a much different starting line. Those who have not yet worked interprofessionally must first develop the foundational skills of group dynamics, effective communication, and conflict resolution. Figure 3.2 illustrates a potential pathway for 3 different clinicians.

It is highly possible that with years of professional experience, a hybrid pathway may be an effective way to blend professional experience with foundational knowledge at a faster pace. Consequently, professional development and continuing education are a personal pathway, and a multitude of factors influence the contour of the road.

Examining the professional standards from the clinical field of practice is a good way to envision what training is needed to practice effective IPCP (see the sidebar Professional Education Standards Related to IPE). In doing so, clinicians are able to evaluate their skills against those of current graduates in the field, highlighting potential strengths and shortfalls in skills. Figure 3.3 presents key words used in the professional standards of 8 health care professions.

SLP and nursing have the most developed framework around IPE, evidenced by the language used across their professional standards that set their curriculum. Of special note, the nursing standards reviewed in figure 3.3 are postprofessional in nature (i.e., for nurses already practicing and achieving their MSN or DNP), whereas the SLP standards guide entry to the profession. Though not an exhaustive list of

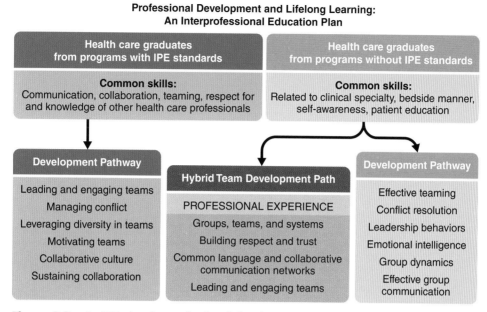

Figure 3.2   An IPE plan for professional development and lifelong learning.

professions, this infographic displays commonalities and differences that exist in the academic topography of IPE that breeds IPCP. These differences may become critical in reflecting on educator readiness to facilitate IPE.

Clinician as IPE Faculty Facilitator

All too often, clinicians are hired to teach in professional and postprofessional health care education programs without any formal teaching preparation. These roles may take the shape of part-time adjunct positions or full-time teaching positions. A clinician with a terminal education degree (PhD, EdD) is scarce in the balance of programs across the United States; furthermore, a PhD does not guarantee teaching experience. Adding to the quandary, health care fields such as PT and OT are graduating students to enter the profession with a terminal degree (i.e., DPT, OTD). Many of these graduates make up the new IPE faculty labor force and serve as clinical educators or fieldwork coordinators in clinical learning environments. Because they have no formal teaching preparation, they teach how they were taught when they were students. This group likely has little clinical experience to draw from, teaching strictly from the book. On top of this challenge, the new graduate may be lucky enough to be hired by a program with an interprofessional thread running through the curriculum. In this case, educator development has to address not only the core elements of effective teaching but also the essentials of IPE as well. This area of IPE is still evolving, and it is expected that over time, competencies will be formed for those teaching IPE and precepting IPCP experiences.[71]

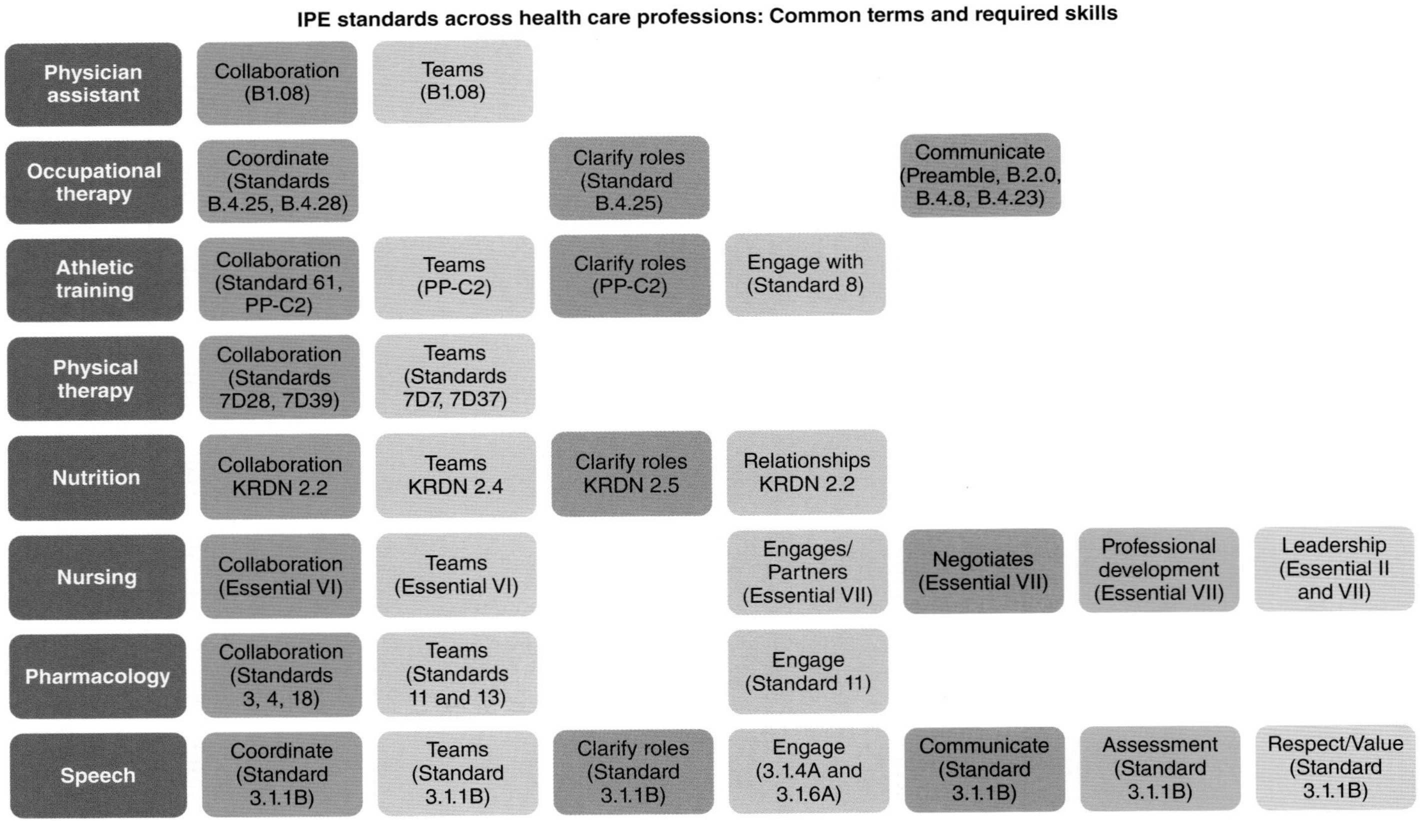

IPE standards across health care professions: Common terms and required skills

Physician assistant	Collaboration (B1.08)	Teams (B1.08)			Communicate (Preamble, B.2.0, B.4.8, B.4.23)		
Occupational therapy	Coordinate (Standards B.4.25, B.4.28)		Clarify roles (Standard B.4.25)				
Athletic training	Collaboration (Standard 61, PP-C2)	Teams (PP-C2)	Clarify roles (PP-C2)	Engage with (Standard 8)			
Physical therapy	Collaboration (Standards 7D28, 7D39)	Teams (Standards 7D7, 7D37)					
Nutrition	Collaboration KRDN 2.2	Teams KRDN 2.4	Clarify roles KRDN 2.5	Relationships KRDN 2.2			
Nursing	Collaboration (Essential VI)	Teams (Essential VI)		Engages/Partners (Essential VII)	Negotiates (Essential VII)	Professional development (Essential VII)	Leadership (Essential II and VII)
Pharmacology	Collaboration (Standards 3, 4, 18)	Teams (Standards 11 and 13)		Engage (Standard 11)			
Speech	Coordinate (Standard 3.1.1B)	Teams (Standard 3.1.1B)	Clarify roles (Standard 3.1.1B)	Engage (3.14A and 3.16A)	Communicate (Standard 3.1.1B)	Assessment (Standard 3.1.1B)	Respect/Value (Standard 3.1.1B)

Figure 3.3 Common terms and required skills in IPE standards across health care professions.

In the National Collaborative for Improving the Clinical Learning Environment (NCICLE) published proceedings that include a categorization of the optimal interprofessional learning environment, optimal environments are characterized by the following six traits[81]:

1. Patient centeredness
2. Continuum of learning
3. Reliable communications
4. Team-based care
5. Shared accountability
6. Evidence-based practice centered on interprofessional care

These categories were fleshed out in prior research,[82] and full descriptions of each category can be found by searching for the report online using the terms "NCICLE Proceedings". The report notes that these categories are shared to promote a team-based care model that can best serve the patient. Clinical sites can also use these categories to begin to evaluate their clinical learning environments for both interns and students from health professions programs. In addition, professional development programs aimed at preparing clinical site instructors and fieldwork educators can use these categories to produce meaningful and impactful training sessions.

Professional Development of the Clinical Preceptor

A gap in the literature exists in the area of preceptor readiness to engage health care students in IPE.[72-76] Additionally, students engaged in clinical education have reported that IPCP doesn't exist at all or is dissimilar to how it is taught in the classroom. This disconnect is likely to result in a lack of forward progress toward global interprofessional health care goals (e.g., Triple Aim, Quadruple Aim) and those of individual professional accrediting bodies. While health care programs are preparing learners for IPCP, they may be failing to prepare their clinical preceptors.[72,76] The limited data that exist on the effectiveness of IPE professional development to foster and assess clinical preceptor preparedness are summarized in chapter 4. However, to begin exploring preceptor development in IPE, the following 10 best practices (based on field experience and evidence from the literature) have been suggested.[78]

1. Set the stage:
   - Provide psychological safety for all participants.
   - Afford the physical space to collaborate.
   - Encourage connections between all participants to learn about each other.
   - Encourage all participants to speak up in collaborations.
2. Model IPCP:
   - Emphasize the value of diverse team members by highlighting their roles.
   - Interprofessional communication should include the learners.
   - Be mindful of all communication and behaviors as the learners are watching.

3. Be aware of professional sensitivities:
   - Consider professional identities (and hierarchy), stereotypes, and cultures.
   - Communicate tactfully; be sensitive to all professions.
4. Keep it centered on the patient:
   - Involve the patient and family with the health care team; acknowledge their roles.
   - Educate the patient and family on team-based care and how it stands to have a positive impact on them.
5. Participate in different interprofessional precepting models:
   - Consider varied models of precepting to accomplish IPCP, including cop-recepting.
   - Implement an interchangeable preceptor model to afford increased exposure to IPCP.
6. Rethink patient presentations:
   - Provide an opportunity for each learner to present the patient at rounds or discussions.
   - Include learner-team presentations where multiple professions collaborate on a presentation.
   - Ensure presentations of cases include all learners and the patient at the bedside or clinic.
7. Ask teaching questions to all learners on the team and facilitate learning:
   - Ask questions of and target discussions toward all learners.
   - Be explicit about collaboration by inviting all learners.
   - Facilitate learner teams to ensure balance across professions.
8. Develop a process for all team members to document:
   - Create an IPCP flow sheet in the health record of the patient.
   - Document the team-based care plan, including professions that contributed.
9. Create a process for reflection and debriefing about IPCP:
   - Be explicit about interprofessional collaboration; make it known that it is a goal.
   - Use IPEC core competencies and subcompetencies as a guide.
10. Develop models of interprofessional evaluation:
    - Use validated tools from the literature to assess IPCP.
    - Revisit the IPEC core competencies and subcompetencies as a guide.
    - Consider using self-evaluations, peer evaluations, and 360° evaluations from all learners and preceptors.

In addition to the above-recommended best practices, a 2019 qualitative study summarized a consensus on interprofessional facilitator capabilities to include the following[80]:

- Incorporating theory and learning frameworks that afford IPE and IPCP
- Maintaining IPE as essential to facilitating IPCP (and behavioral change)

- Managing the learning environment to facilitate IPE and IPCP
- Modeling patient-centered care
- Using common language consistently

Interprofessional precepting is an essential skill needed to provide authentic clinical learning experiences for professional students. This is where the rubber meets the road, where skills are refined that will be practiced by students once they are certified or licensed, and preceptor readiness to facilitate IPCP cannot be assumed. What's more, implementing facilitator training (including the previously suggested best practices) stands to rectify the disparity between what students learn in the classroom and what they experience in the clinical practice setting.[75,78]

Summary

IPE has the potential to improve the efficiency and impact of health care teams. The opportunity to collaborate with health care peers, or teaming, should be present in all IPE professional development models. Learning to function on teams based on roles and responsibilities, becoming aware of and managing stereotypes and biases by learning about health care peers, and understanding one's own leadership and coping styles all inform best practices in teaming (refer to chapter 4 for evidence on best practices). Highly functioning teams are critical to health care, and IPE professional development should be delivered in a model that parallels real-life teams.

Additionally, this chapter presented faculty facilitation as a required skill of effective IPE delivery. Elements of professional development programs for preparing faculty facilitators were discussed, and creating a culture for IPCP was encouraged. Finally, this chapter presented potential pathways for individualized professional development in IPE and IPCP and provided both personal and organizational rationale for growth. Chapter 4 will offer an opportunity to review the depth and breadth of global evidence and how it can influence the planning and facilitation of IPE.

CASE STUDY Debriefing

Joel appears to be practicing athletic training in a silo, or without the help of other health care team members (i.e., Jan, the nurse). At the high school, it is common for the nurse and athletic trainer to provide care for the general student population and the athletes, respectively. Care coordination becomes essential when there is an overlap in roles, such as when athletes suffer from general medical illness or disease (e.g., diabetes management, seizures). However, when an athlete injures a knee or elbow, the athletic trainer may take the lead or handle it completely depending on the skills of the team dyad.

In this case, a staff member was injured, calling both team members into action. Joel failed to alert Jan, deciding to handle it himself. In the future, this decision may prove to be a grave mistake; an amputation displaying shock symptoms is an emergency. Joel was unable to take vitals and stop the bleeding efficiently. He needed a trained health care peer to assist him in care delivery, and care was delayed because he did not alert his team.

To be an effective team member, a clinician must have a positive attitude toward collaboration, be able to negotiate roles on a team, and display behaviors consistent with teamwork (e.g., the ability to lead and follow). Joel portrayed negative body language during communications, disinterest in learning about members on his team, and a general lack of engagement or effort to collaborate with his health care peers.

Standard athletic training protocol calls for an emergency action plan (EAP) for the high school, outlining staff roles for handling emergencies at the various athletic venues. Jan may use this as a communication tool, establishing the idea of a team for Joel; EAPs require regular review and procedural training as a team, affording an opportunity to convene as a group. Joel, and more importantly the patients he provides cares for, are suffering as he refuses to learn from others on his care team.

Foundational elements of effective care teams are trust, respect, and an understanding of KSAs of each profession. In this case, Joel may have no idea what FNPs are or what they are capable of doing in a trauma setting. IPE is a new pedagogy, something Joel was not exposed to in his athletic training education 40 years ago. Professional development on collaborative care plays a role in forming teams, exploring roles on the team, and coordinating efficient care.

Case Study Discussion Questions

1. Joel attempted to handle the trauma situation on his own. How can Jan get Joel to buy into the team approach?
2. Joel may have no idea what Jan and Molly are trained to do. What can they do to educate him on the clinical skills of their profession?
3. When new members join a care team (e.g., Jan), what approaches enable the group to become an efficient team?
4. Suggest a professional development plan for Joel, Jan, and Molly using resources presented in this chapter. How might the plans be different? How might the plans be the same?

CHAPTER 4

Essential Evidence

Judi Schack-Dugré, PT, DPT, MBA, EdD
Jordan Hamson-Utley, PhD, LAT, ATC

Objectives

After reading this chapter, the reader will be able to do the following:

- Understand the areas of current research related to IPE and IPCP.
- Use Kirkpatrick's expanded outcomes typology in the evaluation of IPE and IPCP evidence.
- Synthesize evidence on the effectiveness of IPE and IPCP.
- Identify the gaps in evidence related to IPE and IPCP.
- Apply evidence related to IPE and IPCP in the classroom or workplace.
- Analyze assessment strategies and tools related IPE and IPCP effectiveness.

CASE STUDY Education Segregation

June is an experienced occupational therapy assistant (OTA) faculty member at a health sciences college in the United States. Her college educates OTAs, physical therapist assistants (PTAs), radiology technicians (RTs), and medical technologists (MTs) across 3 campuses. In addition, June's college highlights the importance of IPCP through institutional learning outcomes, which translate to the learning outcomes and resulting coursework for each program. The college has a new dean of health sciences, who shared with June the importance of IPE in the preparation of new providers for today's health care market. This is one of the main reasons June accepted her position at the college—opportunities for IPE abounded!

This week, June attends a meeting where faculty discuss and vote on segregating PTA and OTA students in core courses. After the two sides debate the pros and cons related to shared educational experiences, the faculty members vote to separate the OTA and PTA programs, losing the main conduit for IPE for these student populations. June is beside herself. Why can't her peers see the value of IPE and the opportunities their college system affords?

(continued)

Case Study *(continued)*
___

As June heads back to her office, a PTA faculty member stops her in the hall and says, "Our students need different things, June. This vote is not against you or the OTA program. We just need more in certain areas than your students do."

June, still emotional from the vote, responds by saying, "Anatomy, principles of therapeutic exercise, and wellness are not profession-specific topics and can be effectively delivered across health care professions in a manner that allows students to learn more than content—they learn how other professions implement these concepts in patient care. We've just lost the opportunity to teach these topics through an IPE lens."

Her colleague pauses, then says, "My peers aren't trained to facilitate an IPE classroom, and I'm not trained, so we're better off splitting up students and teaching to what we know is true. OTA guest speakers are not PTAs. OTs and OTAs have not practiced PT, so how can they teach our prelicensed PTA students how to facilitate wellness in our patients? We just can't change the curriculum to accommodate IPE."
___

Understanding negative perceptions of and barriers to IPE and how they affect the advancement of IPE requires further consideration. It is clear that June's colleague (and the faculty members who voted to segregate the professions) would gain from learning about the benefits of IPCP linked with evidence supporting the Quadruple Aim.[1] June's colleague also mentioned something that likely needs to be addressed across existing IPE initiatives: professional development (see chapter 3). The assumption that faculty members understand the evolving roles of providers with increasing specialization and how these unique roles influence team collaboration; value peers outside their discipline; and know how to effectively communicate across health professions must be made with caution. It is apparent that June is ready to facilitate change.

Influence of Faculty

Faculty members have direct influence on IPE outcomes and thus can be a primary edifice supporting IPE. Faculty perceptions of IPE were found to be a key factor in creating meaningful encounters.[2] As in any educational interface, learning is optimized for most individuals when intentional pedagogy is employed. Effective IPE necessitates planned learning activities whereby the faculty member not only is an expert in content but also supports the premise of IPE and its importance to health care delivery.[3] Many faculty members have limited experience and expertise in facilitating IPE and require support.[4] Additionally, many feel unprepared and lack confidence in providing IPE and therefore are resistant to its adoption. This lack of perceived competency can promote negative faculty perceptions of IPE, which then translate to the student experience. Student perceptions of their learning are linked to their perceptions of faculty competency.[5]

There are faculty members within the health professions with expertise in IPE facilitation. The consensus found in the literature is that faculty leaders who are experts in IPE should advocate for its advancement in academic settings. These leaders are **faculty champions** and are necessary for IPE curricula to be successfully developed, implemented, and sustained.[4,6,7] Faculty champions embrace the knowledge and passion to advocate for and facilitate change at their institution or practice setting.

Shaping IPE

IPE became popular when health care was deemed to be in a quality crisis and in need of systematic restructuring to better meet the needs of a progressive society.[8] This redesign of the health care system commanded that academia be an integral component of this effort.[9] Academic and industry leaders in health professions were commissioned to convene and propose an action plan. Academic institutions were to reexamine their curricula and integrate formalized interprofessional learning activities. Ultimately these experiences were to be supported through regulatory mandates of accreditation and processes for professional credentialing.[8]

Deemed the pedagogical strategy of choice for educating health professionals for collaborative team-based health care delivery, IPE was recommended to be included in the educational program of every health profession.[8] Shifting from a siloed, single-discipline education to one involving multiple disciplines working as a team indicated a movement toward IPE.[10] Interprofessional activities that can be accomplished within this type of curriculum have been determined to be effective for changing attitudes toward IPE and collaboration,[11] as well as improving patient outcomes[12] and creating systems change.[13]

The study of IPE dates back only a few decades, and terminology, definitions, and research efforts are still developing. Using a modified version of Kirkpatrick's expanded outcomes typology (figure 4.1),[14] tables 4.1 through 4.6 highlight a sample of existing IPE research as of 2018 using a scoping review across the 6 levels of the typology:

1. Learner's reaction
2a. Change in attitudes and perceptions
2b. Change in knowledge and skills
3. Change in behavior
4a. Change in organizational practice
4b. Benefits to patients, families, and communities

TOOLS OF IPE
Accreditation Dictates the What, Not the How

Despite a lack of consensus regarding accrediting standards across health disciplines and the ambiguity of future directions, IPE continues to be a topic of widespread research within the health professions. In particular, much research has been conducted to better understand the mechanisms to optimally implement and use this preferred pedagogical approach to teaching health professionals.[8] The resource center at Nexus encapsulates the literature and shares strategies for implementation of IPE across disciplines and teaching modalities. Conduct an Internet search for "Nexus IPE Resource Center" to connect with the aforementioned tools for IPE.

The use of scoping reviews to summarize evidence in the field has become increasingly popular in the health sciences.[15] This categorization is beneficial for understanding investigational rigor within the current IPE literature. Although findings from all 6 levels will be summarized, pay particular attention to levels 3, 4a, and 4b; they are considered the target zone for future research.[16]

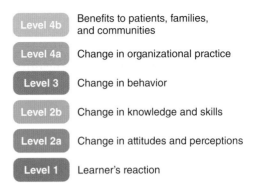

Level 4b	Benefits to patients, families, and communities
Level 4a	Change in organizational practice
Level 3	Change in behavior
Level 2b	Change in knowledge and skills
Level 2a	Change in attitudes and perceptions
Level 1	Learner's reaction

Figure 4.1 Kirkpatrick's expanded outcomes typology.

Taking Aim

Before examining the research associated with each level of Kirkpatrick's typology, it is important to weave in the impact of the Triple Aim and Quadruple Aim on the findings to date. In 2007, the IHI introduced the Triple Aim.[17] This initiative was created with the primary goal of improving population health by improving the health care system in the United States. Guiding health care organizations and providers to improve access, cost, and the patient's experience would meet this goal. The Triple Aim encapsulates 3 interwoven factors (figure 4.2): per capita cost, population health, and patient care experience. To date, much of the IPE and IPCP research aims to assess the elements of the Triple Aim. The IHI purports that the 3 elements must be balanced; an unequal strength in one area will result in a corresponding weakness or shortage in another. For example, if the experience of care is augmented to best-practice levels, the associated cost of this change may affect access to care for some.

Connecting the Triple Aim to Kirkpatrick's typology, cost of care correlates with level 4a, and health outcomes and patient satisfaction correlate with level 4b. However, while these levels (3, 4a, 4b) are the proposed target of current and future research, it is difficult to replicate findings from one study to the next due to environmental differences (e.g., intricacies of health care settings); thus, the evidence on IPE and IPCP effectiveness often lacks strength and remains questionable.

The Quadruple Aim[1] adds an important element to the Triple Aim and the effectiveness of health care systems—the provider experience. The provider experience is characterized by the work life of those providing care across health care settings, including

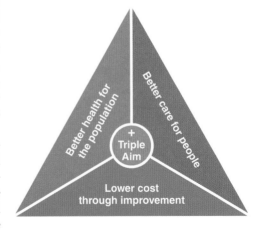

Figure 4.2 Triple Aim.

clinicians and staff. Burnout in health care providers has been correlated with a decrease in patient satisfaction,[18,19] a negative impact on patient health outcomes,[19-21] and an increase in cost to provide care.[22] The Quadruple Aim (figure 4.3) advances the Triple Aim by integrating the provider's satisfaction as an equal element in the optimization of health systems.

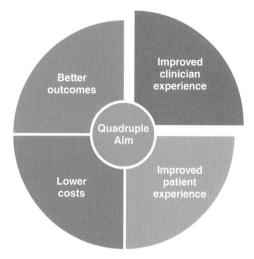

Participants who engage in IPE have been found to benefit in varying ways. Consistent with the 2016 IPEC framework, research has reported that medical and nursing students who engaged in an IPE approach to health care delivery perceived that they had superior collaborative skills compared

Figure 4.3   Quadruple Aim.

with those who did not engage in IPE.[23] Faculty perceptions of enhanced student collaborative skills were also found as a response to IPE.[24]

Evidence has supported a multitude of advantages of IPE[23]:

- The cultivation of mutual respect and trust for each other
- Improved knowledge of professional roles and responsibilities
- Use of effective communication strategies
- Increased job satisfaction
- Improved patient outcomes
- Fewer medical errors

As students engage in IPE, their familiarity with one another and their associated professional roles provides a more comfortable environment for exchanges, thus increasing job satisfaction. As this collective comfort level improves, the sharing of knowledge and care delivery improve.[25]

EBP OF TEAMSHIP
Colocate Teams to Improve Efficiency

Locating physicians in the same physical space as their team members has been shown to improve their efficiency by recovering .5 hour of physician time each day, 2.5 hours per week. This recovered time stands to influence patient-visit capacity (level 4a) and has the potential to decrease practitioner (physician and nonphysician) burnout by empowering nonphysicians to share in patient care (by delegating nonphysician tasks). What's more, colocation may facilitate achievement of the Quadruple Aim.[99]

Connecting the Quadruple Aim to Kirkpatrick's typology, evidence related to the provider's satisfaction corresponds to levels 4a and 4b. At level 4a, the organization might make a change to the work life of the clinician, resulting in less burnout and thereby improving the provider's satisfaction. For example, expanding the role of nurses and medical assistants to operate under a physician's standing orders increases daily workflow and fosters team cohesiveness.[26,27] At level 4b, providers might fight burnout by seeing the fruits of their labors in their recovering patients, families, and communities. In a study of physician burnout, the leading predictor of job satisfaction was being able to provide quality care.[28]

Finally, before summarizing the existing data by level of Kirkpatrick's typology, it is important to explain how the studies were selected for discussion in this chapter. A scoping review was initiated that focused on systematic reviews and summary reports of evidence from IPE and IPCP research over 4 decades. In addition to these reviews and summaries, newly published peer-reviewed literature or gray literature not included in the aforementioned were examined, classified by typology, and reported herein if they offered novel findings or were documented as strong evidence (either positive or negative). As a result, the tables are not exhaustive; however, they encompass a sample of evidence, both positive and negative, across each level of Kirkpatrick's expanded outcomes typology.[14]

Learner's Reaction (Level 1) Evidence

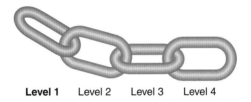

Level 1   Level 2   Level 3   Level 4

The literature is filled with research on IPE; however, the majority of investigations emphasize student perceptions and attitudes toward IPE. Studies on the outcomes of IPE and its ability to change behavior in the workplace are scarce.[29,30] This section of the review will summarize learners' reactions as a result of partaking in IPE or IPCP. These reactions were collected via quantitative and qualitative means and presented in peer-reviewed literature and gray literature. Table 4.1 presents a study that assessed the learners' reactions to IPE. Many of the findings in this area overlap almost entirely; one study is sufficient to portray the value of assessment at this level.

TABLE 4.1   Evidence at Kirkpatrick's Level 1

STUDY AUTHORS: Pfaff, Baxter, Ploeg, and Jack (2014)[100]

Sample size (*n*): 514

Population: Graduate nursing students

Intervention: Curricular infusion, not well described

Measurement tool: Collaborative practice assessment survey; qualitative interview

Findings: Students were satisfied with the IPE experience, teams and team function, and mentorship opportunities; the number of disciplines and accessible faculty, leaders, and managers significantly influenced interprofessional competence and engagement.

IPEC competency: 4

Though it is not the focus of future research, sampling the learner's reaction to IPE can prove useful as a benchmark for first-year students or those encountering IPE or IPCP for the first time. Additionally, it may be obvious from the reported findings that this type of assessment is also useful for program development and refinement, shaping future IPE offerings. However, it has been widely communicated through the literature that this level of assessment (Kirkpatrick level 1) is of little predictive worth in creating change in practice (Kirkpatrick levels 3, 4a, 4b), and assessments at this level are of little use once IPE becomes established.[31]

TOOLS OF IPE
Assessing Level 1

The assessment and evaluation repository at NCIPE has limited the inclusion of tools that assess at this level and placed emphasis on tools that measure skills, behaviors, and system change. The TeamSTEPPS Teamwork Attitudes Questionnaire (T-TAQ) [32] and the W(e) Learn Interprofessional Program Assessment Scale[33] are the only assessments included in this category. Of these, the TeamSTEPPS assessments show high utility because they are stand-alone assessments with acceptable validity and reliability that can be used without full implementation of TeamSTEPPS; they can assess team opinions of an IPE program or a single IPE activity.

Change in Attitudes, Perceptions, Knowledge, and Skills (Level 2) Evidence

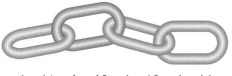

Level 1   **Level 2**   Level 3   Level 4

The literature is replete with data on student perceptions of IPE and their influence. Areas that have been investigated include personal professional identity, other professions' roles and responsibilities, professional hierarchies, communication, teamwork, trust, and IPE in general as an instructional strategy and learning environment. However, there is inconsistency within the literature on the impact of students' perceptions on these various constructs within IPE.

Threats to professional identity have been found to demonstrate a key failure in IPCP[34] and thus are an important target of IPE programming. Researchers found improved professional identities following IPE when the experiences were perceived as relevant to the students' future practice.[35] Evidence also shows that participation in a high-fidelity IPE simulation focusing on roles and responsibilities and communication within a health care team produced improved perceptions of other professions by nursing, OT, and respiratory therapy students.[36] Data on effectiveness of IPE are not always positive; Michalec and colleagues[37] identified conflicting data on student perceptions and attitudes toward IPE whereby some learners experienced a positive change and others found that IPE had little or no impact on student perceptions.

Reduced hierarchal categorization between the health professions was determined to occur following an IPE experience. However, this diminution cannot specifically be related to the IPE program; it may have also been influenced by external interactions of students as a result of their IPE experiences.[37] Results from other studies examining roles and responsibilities and professional identities revealed corroborating data showing that perceptions of other providers' roles improved with IPE contact.[37,38] Moreover, Stull and Blue[39] discovered that an introductory IPE course did not positively affect student attitudes toward other professions but did demonstrate a weakened personal professional identity that was foundational for IPE readiness.

Enhanced perceptions and understanding of interprofessional roles and responsibilities are the basis for improved communication and teamwork. Health care delivery teams that are deficient in their ability to communicate and collaborate within the team can negatively impact patient safety and health outcomes.[40,41] From a fiscal perspective, inefficiencies in provider communication cost U.S. hospitals more than $12.4 billion per year.[41] The results of Granheim and colleagues[40] support the notion that IPE has a positive influence on communication between professions and the realization that collaboration in the workplace is essential. Roberts and colleagues[35] found that students revealed an improved perception of their professional skills in communication and collaboration following IPE. Additionally, the importance and relevance of IPCP were enhanced when students appreciated that future clinical practice would be directly affected by these skills following a large-scale IPE experience.[35,42]

The overarching importance of these referenced data is that students' perceptions guide their engagement, satisfaction, and learning.[43] Perceived usefulness of content, a feeling of autonomy, and faculty support were highly correlated with goal orientation and self-efficacy, which are key constructs for learning.[44] Liaw and colleagues[45] found that students' perceptions toward future IPE learning were improved following an IPE experience. If perceptions of IPE are negative in either students or facilitators, learning is not optimized and translation to clinical practice is hindered. Students' perceptions, knowledge, and skills are the precursor to behavior manifestations and practice change. Table 4.2 presents various research that assessed learners' attitudes, perceptions, knowledge, and skills related to IPE.

TABLE 4.2   Evidence at Kirkpatrick's Level 2a and 2b

STUDY AUTHORS: Hudak, Melcher, and de Oliveira (2017)[88]

Sample size (*n*): 14

Population: PA preceptors from a variety of clinical settings

Intervention: Qualitative data-gathering methodology, including interviews, audio transcription, and thematic coding

Measurement tool: Interview guide and qualitative analysis by NVivo 11; theoretical saturation was met with this sample size

Findings: Four themes emerged:

1. Preceptors define interprofessional practice differently
2. Students learn about terms by being part of teams
3. Preceptors separate students to avoid diluting learning experiences
4. Preceptors can facilitate IPE by introducing students to members of the team and by modeling team skills

IPEC competency: 4

STUDY AUTHORS: Arenson, Umland, Collins et al. (2015)[101]

Sample size (*n*): 577

Population: Undergraduate students in nursing, medicine, PT, OT, pharmacy, and counseling

Intervention: A total of 4 team interactions over 2 years with volunteer patients

Measurement tool: Self- and peer teamwork evaluation

Findings: Value of and respect for other professions, attitudes toward team-based patient care, and understanding of patient's perspective all improved.

IPEC competency: 1, 4

STUDY AUTHORS: Bates, Mellin, Paluta, Anderson-Butcher, Vogeler, and Sterling (2019)[102]

Sample size (*n*): 27 interviewees; 340 students

Population: CARE (consultation, assessment, referral, and education) teams made up of health care and nonhealth-related professions, including mental health clinicians, psychologists, community mental health therapists, and intervention specialists, in Title I elementary schools in the Western United States

Intervention: Structured activities for CARE team members to learn how to assess and refer students for intervention within the team, how to communicate with parents and caregivers, and how to work together to set and align goals for student success

Measurement tool: Team processes based on the systems of care model from the University of Maryland's National Center for School Mental Health; monthly monitoring of outcomes; interviews with 27 CARE team members from 4 schools

Findings: CARE team processes improved access to services and consistency of follow-through on plans and interventions. Additionally, academic, behavioral, and mental health outcomes markedly improved in students identified as having challenges in these areas. Increased knowledge of strategies, interventions, resources, and support systems was reported by CARE team members.

IPEC competency: 2, 3, 4

STUDY AUTHORS: Berg, Wong, and Vincent (2010)[103]

Sample size (n): 16

Population: Undergraduate students in medicine and nursing

Intervention: SBAR IPE training using online, remote manikin simulation

Measurement tool: Checklist of observed communication strategies for during and after simulation used by remote instructor

Findings: Student communication skills improved.

IPEC competency: 3

STUDY AUTHORS: Brashers, Haizlip, and Owen (2019)[84]

Sample size (n): 113

Population: A total of 28 teams made up of faculty and clinicians, with each team consisting of 3 to 7 participants from at least 2 professions from multiple institutions

Intervention: Semiannual IPE development program held at UVA (University of Virginia) for 3.5 days between November 2015 and November 2017 using the ASPIRE model as a framework for a curriculum to instruct faculty and clinicians from across the country in developing IPE activities at all levels of postsecondary training, including in the workplace

Measurement tool: Web-based surveys

Findings: The ASPIRE model can be an effective training framework for developing IPE opportunities in postsecondary environments.

IPEC competency: 1, 2, 3, 4

STUDY AUTHORS: Cartwright, Franklin, Forman et al. (2013)[134]

Sample size (n): 125

Population: Undergraduate students in nursing, OT, social work, speech pathology, and health information management

Intervention: Asynchronous IPE in groups on dementia case

Measurement tool: Pre- and postintervention Interprofessional Socialization and Valuing Scale (ISVS-21)

Findings: Significant positive change was found in the ISVS-21 grand mean; only 42 students completed both pre- and posttest surveys.

IPEC competency: 1, 2, 3, 4

STUDY AUTHORS: Coleman, Roberts, Wulff, van Zyl, and Newton (2008)[135]

Sample size (n): 56

Population: Graduate students in nursing, medicine, and social work

Intervention: Weekly collaborative patient care and monthly collaborative learning over 1 year

Measurement tool: Pre- and posttest self-assessment of attitudes, knowledge, skills, and competence

Findings: Improvements were shown in collaboration, valuing interprofessional teams, conflict resolution, and patient care roles on IPCP teams.

IPEC competency: 1, 2, 4

STUDY AUTHORS: Curran, Sharpe, Flynn, and Button (2010)[136]

Sample size (*n*): 1,206

Population: Undergraduate students in nursing, medicine, pharmacy, and social work

Intervention: Case-based 2-week patient simulations, 3 per year over 3 years

Measurement tool: Self-assessment of attitudes (IPE and teamwork) and satisfaction with learning mode

Findings: No significant change was found in positive attitudes toward IPCP (teamwork) or IPE; significant differences existed between professions.

IPEC competency: 4

STUDY AUTHORS: Dallaghan, Hultquist, Nickol et al. (2018)[137]

Sample size (*n*): 175

Population: Health science students in allied health, medicine, nursing, pharmacy, and public health

Intervention: Baseline scores on NIPEAS-19 collected from students' first term during a dedicated IPE day; follow-up data collected 2 years later following an IPE event

Measurement tool: NIPEAS 19-item Likert scale questionnaire that assesses attitudes toward IPE; based on IPEC competencies; designed for longitudinal study design

Findings: A significant increase in positive attitudes toward IPE was sampled at the 2-year follow-up, with all but nursing (*n* = 24) and public health (*n* = 3) students showing positive change.

IPEC competency: 1, 2, 3, 4

STUDY AUTHORS: Dahlgren, Gibbs, Greenwalt et al. (2018)[10]

Sample size (*n*): 278

Population: Graduate and postlicense students in nursing, pharmacy, OT, and PT

Intervention: IPE orientation focused on roles and responsibilities of health care peers

Measurement tool: RIPLS pre- and posttest design

Findings: Significant changes in attitudes toward roles of health care peers were achieved following a 2-hour IPE orientation, except for one question on the RIPLS that addressed the need for acquiring more skills than others.

IPEC competency: 2

STUDY AUTHORS: Iachini, DeHart, Browne et al. (2018)[138]

Sample size (*n*): 30

Population: Graduate and undergraduate students in pharmacy, social work, public health, and business

Intervention: Examining the impact of implementing a collaborative leadership model within IPE on students' perceptions of leadership on health care teams

Measurement tool: Pre- and posttest survey design examining SCM (social change model) and leadership efficacy; qualitative interviews at course poster sessions

Findings: Students significantly improved their perceptions of leadership efficacy; findings also indicated improvements in 3 group-level values of the SCM: collaboration, common purpose, and controversy with civility. Overall conclusions from qualitative data include students learning to view leadership as a collaborative team process and more of a process than a role; implications for IPE were shared.

IPEC competency: 4

STUDY AUTHORS: Kenaszchuk, Rykhoff, Collins et al. (2012)[139]

Sample size (*n*): 131

Population: Undergraduate and graduate students in nursing, funeral services, pharmacy, OTA, PTA, paramedics, and social work

Intervention: Large-group 3-hour workshop with lecture and case-based learning

Measurement tool: Pre- and postworkshop self-assessment survey

Findings: Large-group IPE can facilitate attitude change regarding teamwork, roles, and IPCP competency; professional experience influenced the effects of the workshops (larger mean change).

IPEC competency: 2, 3, 4

STUDY AUTHORS: McFadyen, Webster, MacLaren, and O'Neill (2010)[140]

Sample size (*n*): 573

Population: Undergraduate students in nursing, PT, OT, podiatry (prosthetics and orthotics), and radiography

Intervention: Intervention group (*n* = 313) experienced IPE weekly for 3 hours, 24 per year over 4 years; control group (*n* = 260)

Measurement tool: Biannual self-assessment of attitudes toward and perceptions of IPE

Findings: Overall, IPE was correlated with a negative shift in attitudes toward teamwork, collaboration, and professional identity. The intervention group did make positive gains in IPE competency and autonomy and showed differences between professions regarding the need for collaboration.

IPEC competency: 4

STUDY AUTHORS: McLeod, Curran, Dumont et al. (2014)[141]

Sample size (*n*): 210

Population: Undergraduate students in nursing, medicine, social work, psychology, and spiritual care

Intervention: E-learning IPE module with synchronous and asynchronous elements

Measurement tool: Survey assessing change in knowledge and attitudes associated with IPE and IPCP

Findings: Significant difference was found in knowledge and attitudes regarding IPE and IPCP, specifically understanding that professional culture varies across professions, understanding the roles of other professions, being comfortable interacting with interprofessional peers, and understanding the need for improving their interprofessional effectiveness.

IPEC competency: 1, 2, 3, 4

STUDY AUTHORS: Packard, Ryan-Haddad, Monaghan, Doll, and Qi (2016)[142]

Sample size (*n*): 666

Population: Undergraduate students in nursing, medicine, PT, OT, pharmacy, dental, social work, EMS (emergency medical services), and allied health

Intervention: Single (*n* = 604) or semester-long (*n* = 62) IPE team service

Measurement tool: Self-assessment postintervention on team skills and perceptions of IPE

Findings: Across groups, significant improvement was found in team skills and positive perceptions of IPE; perceptions of teaming were more positive in the longitudinal group (*n* = 62).

IPEC competency: 4

STUDY AUTHORS: Pollard and Miers (2008)[143]

Sample size (*n*): 414

Population: Graduate students in nursing, PT, OT, midwifery, radiotherapy, and social work

Intervention: Intervention group (*n* = 275) experienced IPE modules assessed in preceptor-supervised practice over 3 years; control group (*n* = 139)

Measurement tool: Self-assessment questionnaire including teamwork skills, attitudes toward IPE, quality of IPCP experiences, and relationships

Findings: Intervention group scored higher on communication confidence, IPCP interactions, and value of interprofessional relationships; age and previous graduate education had a more negative impact on scores.

IPEC competency: 1, 4

STUDY AUTHORS: Pollard, Miers, and Rickaby (2012)[144]

Sample size (*n*): 29

Population: Graduate students in nursing, midwifery, and social work

Intervention: Intervention group (*n* = 19) experienced IPE modules assessed in preceptor-supervised practice over 3 years; control group (*n* = 10)

Measurement tool: Qualitative interview

Findings: Intervention group reflections included more complex understanding of IPCP roles, teamwork, and communication related to teaming.

IPEC competency: 2, 3, 4

STUDY AUTHORS: Quesnelle, Bright, and Salvati (2018)[145]

Sample size (*n*): 90

Population: Medical and pharmacy students; 12 groups of 6 medical and 2 pharmacy students each

Intervention: Simulated telehealth collaboration; 60-minute large-group case study discussion; 30-minute interprofessional groups debrief, 30-minute intraprofessional debrief using Google Hangout

Measurement tool: Pre- and posttest survey design completed by 90 of 96 students to assess 4 domains: responsibility and accountability, shared authority, IPE, and pharmacogenomics

Findings: Study findings include a significant improvement across all areas of IPCP; medical students' knowledge increased significantly following IPE, albeit with education from their pharmacy student peers.

IPEC competency: 2, 4

STUDY AUTHORS: Rens and Joosten (2014)[146]

Sample size (*n*): 32

Population: Graduate students in OT and teachers

Intervention: Four 7-week fieldwork placements as part of curriculum

Measurement tool: Questionnaire; focus groups

Findings: OTs should spend more time in school to learn routines and obstacles; build relationships with teachers to understand roles and build equal partnerships in collaborative decision making; and involve parents in collaborative decision making.

IPEC competency: 1, 2

STUDY AUTHORS: Shoemaker, deVoest, Booth et al. (2015)[147]

Sample size (*n*): 72

Population: Graduate students in pharmacy, PA, and PT

Intervention: Intervention group (*n* = 34) experienced interprofessional team working on virtual patient case; control group (*n* = 38) received didactic information only

Measurement tool: IPEC competency survey and RIPLS pre- and postintervention assessment

Findings: Intervention group showed significant improvement on several IPEC and RIPLS questions as a result of teamwork on a virtual patient case. IPEC questions measured communication, confidence, and collaboration; RIPLS questions measured professional identity, teamwork, collaboration, roles, and responsibility.

IPEC competency: 2, 3, 4

STUDY AUTHORS: Shrader, Kostoff, Shin et al. (2016)[148]

Sample size (*n*): 163

Population: Nursing, medicine, pharmacy, OT, and dietitian students

Intervention: Communication using SBAR via telephone for medication therapy management; online transition of care

Measurement tool: Interprofessional communication; Attitudes Toward Health Care Teams Scale (ATHCTS) pre- and postsurvey to measure the impact of communication simulation on students' attitudes, confidence, and performance related to IPCP communication and collaboration

Findings: Significant positive change was found in 5 of 20 ATHCTS questions.

IPEC competency: 3

STUDY AUTHORS: Solomon and Geddes (2010)[149]

Sample size (*n*): 11

Population: Undergraduate students in nursing, medicine, OT, and physiotherapy

Intervention: Asynchronous online IPE learning modules

Measurement tool: Assessing students learning with, about, and from each other using online modalities via interview and focus group

Findings: Qualitative results revealed online learning is effective for learning about health care roles.

IPEC competency: 2

STUDY AUTHORS: Soubra, Badr, Zahran et al. (2018)[38]

Sample size (*n*): 266

Population: Senior-level prelicensed students (*n* = 266) in nursing (*n* = 12), medicine (*n* = 47), dentistry (*n* = 39), medical lab technology (*n* = 36), nutrition and dietetics (*n* = 27), pharmacy (*n* = 75), and physical therapy (*n* = 30)

Intervention: Program consisting of 2 sessions (2 hours long each) introducing basic skills for team collaboration (phase 1), case study on roles and responsibilities (phase 2), collaborative group work on patient care planning (phase 3), and development of patient education materials in interprofessional care teams (phase 4)

Measurement tool: Faculty-graded coursework of student intraprofessional and interprofessional teams using standardized rubric

Findings: No significant difference was found between individual and intraprofessional team scores on roles and patient-care planning coursework; students on interprofessional teams scored significantly higher on roles and care planning in comparison to students on intraprofessional teams.

IPEC competency: 2

STUDY AUTHORS: Stull and Blue (2016)[39]

Sample size (*n*): 864

Population: First-year undergraduate students in nursing (*n* = 129), medicine (*n* = 230), pharmacy (*n* = 160), OT (*n* = 47), clinical laboratory science (*n* = 66), dentistry (*n* = 98), dental hygiene (*n* = 24), dental therapy (*n* = 10), public health (*n* = 1), and veterinary medicine (*n* = 100)

Intervention: Participation in a semester-long IPE course, Foundations of Interprofessional Communication and Collaboration (FIPCC), that met on Fridays for 2.5 hours

Measurement tool: Pre- and posttest RIPLS; Interdisciplinary Education Perception Scale (IEPS)

Findings: Student attitudes toward their own and other professions declined; positive correlation was shown between a weakened professional identity and readiness for IPE. This study found that an introductory IPE course did not positively affect student attitudes toward other professions or strengthen professional identity or readiness for interprofessional learning.

IPEC competency: 1, 3, 4

STUDY AUTHORS: Sytsma, Haller, Youdas et al. (2015)[150]

Sample size (*n*): 41

Population: Undergraduate students in medicine and PT

Intervention: A total of 2 peer-teaching dissection sessions using case-based IPE

Measurement tool: IPE curriculum survey

Findings: Significant difference between professions was shown in valued and desired opportunity to learn about another profession, increased role clarity with IPCP (medicine), and decreased value of IPE (PT).

IPEC competency: 1, 2

STUDY AUTHORS: Wellmon, Gilin, Knauss et al. (2012)[104]

Sample size (*n*): 123

Population: Undergraduate students in education, psychology, PT, and social work

Intervention: Large-group workshop with both interprofessional and uniprofessional activities using case-based planning

Measurement tool: Pre- and postworkshop self-assessment of knowledge and attitudes

Findings: Large-group IPE can lead to improved knowledge and attitudes regarding IPCP roles and collaboration; profession and age influenced student responses.

IPEC competency: 2, 4

STUDY AUTHORS: Zaudke, Chestnut, Paolo, and Schrader (2016)[77]

Sample size (*n*): 64

Population: Undergraduate students in nursing, medicine, and pharmacy

Intervention: IPE teamwork teaching (.5 day) and IPCP patient care (2.5 days) over 4 or 8 weeks

Measurement tool: Peer and faculty teamwork assessment using Interprofessional Teaching Objective Structured Clinical Examination (iTOSCE)

Findings: Faculty ratings of teamwork behaviors were higher (20%) compared with peer ratings (8%). Communication scores increased; however, they were the lowest rated for both peer and faculty.

IPEC competency: 4

STUDY AUTHORS: Zanotti, Sartor, and Canova (2015)[151]

Sample size (*n*): 277

Population: Second-year medical students (Italy)

Intervention: Training infused into curriculum

Measurement tool: Pre- and posttest IEPS

Findings: Statistically significant improvements were found in students' overall attitudes as measured by IEPS and 4 subscale scores. Gender (female) and having a family member practicing medicine had a negative impact on change scores. Results indicate that IPE training has a positive influence on students' understanding of collaboration and improved attitudes in interprofessional teamwork.

IPEC competency: 4

COLLABORATIVE CORNER
Multi-Institutional IPE

A common barrier to IPE is geography, be it proximity or presence. Many programs for health professions exist at small schools where they may be the only profession represented. Conversely, many larger schools have multiple health professions on campus, but they may not be physically close enough to share instructional space. Often the key to success is thinking outside the box, and that holds true when cultivating an IPE effort. Think about networking with other institutions at conferences or via social media (e.g., LinkedIn) to find like-minded people who may be facing similar IPE barriers. Then, consider creating a curriculum that can be offered online, synchronously or asynchronously, or even in a blended fashion if geography affords a face-to-face session or two across the semester. Finally, it must make sense, meaning the professions that connect on the effort should afford real-life exposure for students entering those professions; they should collaborate with, and learn about and from, those with whom they will be practicing.

Behavioral Change (Level 3) Evidence

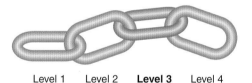

Level 1   Level 2   **Level 3**   Level 4

Definitive evidence linking IPE to desirable intermediate and final outcomes does not yet exist. A study of the evidence on the effectiveness of IPE begins in the classroom and ends at the patient's bedside. Today, those preparing to enter a health care profession are taught not only the skills of their trade but also how to function on an interprofessional care team. These skills might include team building, communicating across disciplines, respecting peer professions, and understanding the various roles and responsibilities of team members.[53] This has been largely influenced by accrediting bodies mandating the inclusion of IPE in professional education (see chapter 3); however, some remain skeptical that IPE is effective in changing behaviors at the bedside. Is there enough evidence?

EBP OF TEAMSHIP
Can Accreditors Drive Change With Mandated IPE?

Zorek and Raehl investigated accreditation directives for IPE in U.S. academic programs offering degrees in dentistry, medicine, nursing, OT, pharmacy, OT, PA, psychology, public health, and social work. Their conclusions suggested that academic accreditation authorities have not put forth a collective initiative to require consistent, explicit IPE norms that must be satisfied in the education of future professionals across all disciplines. This lack of consistency in IPE characterization, use, and implementation leaves the path forward somewhat ambiguous for acculturating IPE into health professions education and ultimately into unified accreditation benchmarks. Regardless of the future trajectory, a common U.S. accreditation standard for all health professions' academic programs would optimize the ability of IPE to transform IPCP[105] as envisioned by WHO.[54]

Although accreditors across the health professions are mandating the inclusion of IPE in professional education (see the Professional Education Standards Related to IPE sidebar in chapter 3), is this enough to create change in practice? What other factors affect the application of what the student has learned in the classroom? Consider the proverb that actions speak louder than words. Current IPE literature suggests that students observe the behaviors and practice patterns of those they shadow while on clinical rotations.[55] Literature also suggests that IPCP may have setting-specific barriers or limitations that affect the application of IPE and IPCP.[23] The gap in findings on the effectiveness of IPE on practice behaviors and system change is likely a main barrier to forward momentum.

Level 3 evidence elucidates the transfer of IPE to clinical practice. Although it can be assessed using many designs, Pollard, Miers, and Gilchrist[56] used a longitudinal approach assessing at 4 time points, including upon entry to the program, after completion of the second year, upon licensure, and at 9 months postlicensure. Though it is difficult to stay connected with students postlicensure, the transfer of IPE to practice is truly assessed in this design. To examine the level 3 evidence further, table 4.3 presents various research that assessed the learners' behavioral change as a result of participating in IPE or IPCP.

TABLE 4.3   Evidence at Kirkpatrick's Level 3

STUDY AUTHORS: Cooke, Chew, Boggis et al. (2003)[106]

Sample size (*n*): 34

Population: Undergraduate students in nursing and medicine

Intervention: Integrative training course for medical and nursing students in breaking bad news to patients

Measurement tool: Triangulation of qualitative methods to gather student perspectives on this experience

Findings: Nursing students were often passive at first (focus-group data indicated they were uncertain of their role), but "from direct observations of the nursing students in our study, we found that they gradually seemed more comfortable interjecting, particularly if they felt they could better explain something to the patient."[106(p141)]

IPEC competency: 2, 3

STUDY AUTHORS: McCutcheon, Whitcomb, Cox, et al. (2017)[85]

Sample size (*n*): 23

Population: Pharmacy preceptors who train health care students in the clinical setting

Intervention: Interprofessional objective structured teaching exercise (iOSTE)

Measurement tool: Survey assessing perceived importance of IPEC core competencies and perceived confidence in precepting students from other health care professions

Findings: A pre- and posttest comparison revealed significant differences in preceptor confidence in teaching interprofessionally ($p = .004$), facilitating an interprofessional simulation debriefing ($p < .001$), conducting the debriefing ($p < .001$), and discussing IPEC core competencies with students ($p = .001$). Additionally, a rubric was used to quantify the behaviors of the preceptor following iOSTE training.

IPEC competency: 1, 2, 3, 4

STUDY AUTHORS: Kilminster and Roberts (2004)[112]

Sample size (*n*): 28

Population: Undergraduate students in nursing ($n = 10$), medicine ($n = 6$), and pharmacy ($n = 12$) at the University of Leeds

Intervention: A pilot IPE project of three 3-hour workshops intended to develop participants' understanding about each other's professional roles, to enhance teaming, and to improve communication skills

Measurement tool: Qualitative interview (1:1)

Findings: Participants emphasized communication skills (both with other professionals and patients) and the development of increased awareness of others' roles; nurses, pharmacists, and doctors reported that the training had an effect on their daily practice. Participants reported increased respect for other professions and improved professional relationships as a result of the workshops.

IPEC competency: 3

STUDY AUTHORS: Morey, Simon, Jay et al. (2002)[113]

Sample size (*n*): 684

Population: Physicians, nurses, and technicians from 9 teaching and community hospital emergency departments (EDs)

Intervention: Emergency Team Coordination Course (ETCC) and implemented formal teamwork structures and processes

Measurement tool: Assessments prior to training and at intervals of 4 and 8 months after training to evaluate 3 outcome constructs (team behavior, ED performance, attitudes and opinions), in which trained observers rated ED team behaviors and made observations of clinical errors, a measure of ED performance; surveys of ED staff and patients measuring attitudes and opinions

Findings: A statistically significant improvement in quality of team behaviors was shown between the experimental and control groups following training ($p = .012$). Subjective workload was not affected by the intervention ($p = .668$). The clinical error rate significantly decreased from 30.9% to 4.4% in the experimental group ($p = .039$). In the experimental group, the ED staff members' attitudes toward teamwork increased ($p = .047$), and staff assessments of institutional support showed a significant increase ($p = .040$).

IPEC competency: 3, 4

STUDY AUTHORS: Mu, Chao, Jensen et al. (2004)[114]

Sample size (*n*): 111

Population: Undergraduate students in OT, PT, and pharmacy

Intervention: Student team collaboration for care on reservations for underserved populations during a 3-year project under faculty supervision

Measurement tool: Pre- and posttest IEPS, 18 items divided into 4 subscales: competency and autonomy, perceived need for cooperation, perception of actual cooperation, and understanding others' value

Findings: Positive perceptions of interprofessional practice significantly increased after project participation; there was a significant impact on length of exposure (participation repetitions), with those who participated having more positive perceptions.

IPEC competency: 4

STUDY AUTHORS: Olander, Coates, Brook et al. (2018)[96]

Sample size (*n*): 18

Population: Midwives, nurses, dietitians, general practitioner, and breastfeeding specialist

Intervention: Interprofessional workshops targeting collaboration between health care providers who care for women before and after pregnancy

Measurement tool: Pre- and posttest; follow-up interview 2 months after workshop to explore changes in practice

Findings: Workshop attendance improved overall attitudes toward collaboration; qualitative follow-up ($n = 12$) revealed several examples of IPCP attributed to workshop attendance.

IPEC competency: 4

STUDY AUTHORS: Pollard, Miers, Gilchrist. (2005)[56]

Sample size (*n*): 723

Population: Undergraduate and graduate students in nursing, OT, PT, radiotherapy, midwifery, mental health, and social work

Intervention: IPE dispersed across curriculum

Measurement tool: Questionnaires concerning communication and teamwork skills and interprofessional learning and working: the University of the West of England (UWE) Entry-Level Interprofessional Questionnaire (ELIQ), the Interim Interprofessional Questionnaire (IIQ), and the Final Interprofessional Questionnaire (FIQ); data collection occurred upon entry to a professional program (baseline data), after completion of the second-year interprofessional module (interim data), upon qualification (qualifying data), and after 9 months of practice as a qualified health or social care professional (practice data)

Findings: Overall results were positive; mature students' responses were more positive than those of younger students. The emergence of differences in responses based on a professional program suggests that IPE may not necessarily influence professional socialization. Demographic and professional variables affecting students' responses in their second year of study demonstrate the complexity of student learning.

IPEC competency: 3, 4

STUDY AUTHORS: Ralyea (2013)[74]

Sample size (*n*): Unknown

Population: Labor and delivery department staff

Intervention: TeamSTEPPS training

Measurement tool: Quality outcomes on labor and delivery, with observations made 6 months following the training; monitoring of metrics such as patient's perception of teamwork, patient's perception of overall quality of work, patient's perception of likelihood to recommend, and employee engagements

Findings: Each metric demonstrated improvements 6 months following TeamSTEPPS training. The participants reported improvements in team structure, leadership, situation monitoring, mutual support, and communication.

IPEC competency: 2, 4

STUDY AUTHORS: Rotz, Dueñas, Zanoni et al. (2016)[75]

Sample size (*n*): 144

Population: Undergraduate students in medicine and pharmacy

Intervention: Interprofessional experiential 6-semester course series wherein 48 student teams (with at least 1 pharmacy student per team) were given 20 minutes to review information about the standardized patient, identify issues that affect the patient's health care, and develop a care plan for the patient

Measurement tool: Student Perceptions of Interprofessional Clinical Education (SPICE), a standardized objective behavioral assessment developed to measure team performance of interprofessional communication and teamwork; Performance Assessment for Communication and Teamwork (PACT-novice)

Findings: A majority of teams demonstrated appropriate competence with respect to interprofessional communication and teamwork. Additionally, a majority of students expressed positive perceptions of IPCP with respect to teamwork, roles and responsibilities, and patient outcomes.

IPEC competency: 1, 2, 3, 4

STUDY AUTHORS: Seaman, Saunders, Dugmore et al. (2018)[97]

Sample size (*n*): 62

Population: Senior-level nursing and medical students

Intervention: Preceptor-supervised interprofessional clinical placement in ambulatory care unit

Measurement tool: ISVS-24 pre- and posttest with qualitative interview

Findings: Overall scores on the ISVS-24 increased significantly after IPE clinical placement; nursing students showed a greater change in scores after placement.

IPEC competency: 1, 2, 3, 4

STUDY AUTHORS: Shiyanbola, Randall, Lammers, Hegge, and Anderson (2014)[70]

Sample size (*n*): 38

Population: Undergraduate students in nursing, medicine, nutrition, pharmacy, and dental hygiene

Intervention: A total of 6 monthly 1- to 2-hour educational workshops with a focus on underserved patients with diabetes

Measurement tool: Clinical diabetes outcomes; patient survey of knowledge and behaviors; student survey of diabetes knowledge and IPCP

Findings: Significant improvement was shown in patient knowledge regarding diabetes (4b), clinical outcomes, and self-management techniques. Students' ability to educate patients significantly increased, as did their awareness of roles on IPCP teams.

IPEC competency: 3, 4

STUDY AUTHORS: Wilhelmsson, Svensson, Timpka, and Faresjö (2013)[152]

Sample size (*n*): 297

Population: Graduate nursing students

Intervention: Intervention group (*n* = 179) experienced 12 weeks of infused IPE curriculum and 2 weeks on clinical rotation on an interprofessional student team; control group (*n* = 118)

Measurement tool: Questionnaire assessing academic preparation for IPCP practice goals

Findings: Intervention group members valued leadership more and were significantly better prepared for their role as nurses, collaborative care, and communication with patients. No difference in perceived preparation for acute patient care was found.

IPEC competency: 1, 3, 4

STUDY AUTHORS: Zaudke, Chestnut, Paolo et al. (2016)[77]

Sample size (*n*): 48

Population: Undergraduate students in nursing, medicine, and pharmacy

Intervention: iTOSCE using a standardized patient developed to assess student IPCP behaviors before and after exposure to the IPE experience; 16 teams with 3 interprofessional members

Measurement tool: Rubric completed by faculty and peer observers to evaluate student teams during the iTOSCE

Findings: Paired *t*-tests demonstrated that both faculty and student ratings of these teams were significantly higher posttest than pretest. A significant interaction revealed that faculty ratings improved more than student ratings from pre- to posttest.

IPEC competency: 3, 4

Organizational Change and Benefits to Patients (Level 4) Evidence

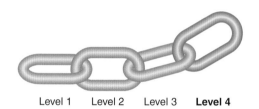

Level 1   Level 2   Level 3   **Level 4**

The benefactor base broadens as the professional identities of the individual student develop: professionals, health care teams, organizations, and patients all benefit. As the characteristics of the chosen profession become more solidified within the individual, understanding of discipline-specific roles and responsibilities of other providers also evolves with IPE.[36,66] As these constructs advance, the team becomes more proficient.[25] Efficient teams develop consensus, participate in effective decision making, are proficient in conflict management, develop trust relationships, and use participative leadership strategies.[67] Thus, ineffective teamwork can place patients at risk.[68] With improved team efficiency, patient outcomes can be optimized, and job satisfaction within the team improves.

Cultivating an environment for the development and sustainability of a high-functioning team benefits the organization as well as the patient. As organizations improve in health care delivery, the overarching system becomes more efficient, benefiting society at large. In an unprecedented study in Japan, Goto and colleagues[69] determined that IPCP was integral in promoting quality-of-life options during the advanced aging stages due to the efficiencies that could be leveraged with improved collaborative health delivery. From these data, it has been shared that the benefactors extend beyond the individual student and collective team of students to include the involved professions, health care organization, and society as a whole.

Potentially the most convincing, exemplary level 4b evidence comes from work by Shiyanbol and colleagues.[70] A diabetes management program for an underserved population led by interprofessional student teams (nursing, medicine, pharmacy, dental hygiene, and nutrition) showed significant improvements in patients' diabetes knowledge, management behaviors, and clinical outcomes. In addition, the study reported student gains in IPEC domains 2 and 3 (roles and responsibilities, communication). The students learned while on teams that were the same or similar to ones they would be on after licensing. What's more, this model is replicable across health professions education and can be implemented through service learning or similar opportunities. Table 4.4 presents various research that assessed changes at the organizational level and patient outcomes as a result of participating in IPE or IPCP.

TABLE 4.4   Evidence at Kirkpatrick's Level 4a and 4b

STUDY AUTHORS: Brewer and Stewart-Wynne (2013)[78]

Sample size (n): 79

Population: Undergraduate students in nursing, medicine, pharmacy, and allied health

Intervention: On-site training for 2 to 3 weeks

Measurement tool: Faculty observation; pre- and posttest self-assessment; client satisfaction survey

Findings: Faculty graded students good to excellent on collaborative competencies (communication rated highest); self-ratings were good to excellent on the IPE experience (level 1 typology). High levels of patient satisfaction were reported.

IPEC competency: 2, 3, 4

STUDY AUTHORS: Dachtyl and Morales (2017)[153]

Sample size (n): 165

Population: Postconcussion K12 students referred to the Cognitive Return to Exertion (CoRTEx) program

Intervention: Academic management team assigned to a student postconcussion and followed through until full return to learn, with a focus on 504 plans, communication strategies, and early intervention

Measurement tool: Qualitative parent and student interview

Findings: Parent and student feedback on CoRTEx was overwhelmingly positive. A point of contact at the school was highlighted as invaluable to parents; coordination of communication regarding the return to the classroom was a great feature; no data reported on student academic outcomes were shared.

IPEC competency: 1, 2, 3, 4

STUDY AUTHORS: Dienst and Byl (1981)[13]

Sample size (*n*): Unknown

Population: Interprofessional undergraduate student teams undertaking community clerkships in nursing, medicine, and pharmacy

Intervention: Community clerkships with 3-member student teams (nursing, medicine, and pharmacy)

Measurement tool: Quality indicators (QIs; teamwork, collaborative problem solving)

Findings: The team education program increased the volume of patients seen (level 4a) and the comprehensiveness of patient care (level 4b).

IPEC competency: 3, 4

STUDY AUTHORS: Congdon and Cate (2019)[86]

Sample size (*n*): Not reported

Population: Fourth-year pharmacy students, RN to BSN students, DNP and FNP students, bachelor and master of social work (BSW and MSW) students

Intervention: Implementation of an IPE clinic flow sheet to organize students' collaboration and communication during patient care

Measurement tool: Multiple surveys using a traditional pre- and posttest methodology (Team Skills Scale [TSS], IPEC Competency Survey, modified ICAR)

Findings: Only TSS findings were reported. The flow sheet had a significant effect on 9 of 17 student perceptions of their behaviors during patient care:

1. Differentiating between contributions based on health care profession
2. Applying professional knowledge in a team care setting
3. Cooperating among disciplines
4. Carrying out responsibilities related to own discipline
5. Communicating during interdisciplinary meetings
6. Adjusting care to support team goals
7. Developing strategies to help patients reach their goals
8. Bringing concerns to team meetings
9. Promoting involvement of team care members who are not participating

IPEC competency: 2, 3, 4

STUDY AUTHORS: Hallin, Henriksson, Dalén, and Kiessling (2011)[79]

Sample size (*n*): 146

Population: Undergraduate students in nursing, medicine, PT, and OT

Intervention: Intervention group (*n* = 84) experienced 2-week clinical IPCP rotation; control group (*n* = 62)

Measurement tool: Patient satisfaction survey at discharge

Findings: Patients in the intervention group reported significantly higher satisfaction with patient education, collaborative decision making, and holistic care (integrating home-life information) as compared with controls.

IPEC competency: 3

STUDY AUTHORS: Walker, Cavallario, Welch-Bacon, Bay, and Van Lunen (2018)[87]

Sample size (*n*): 58 students; 1,319 patient encounters (PE) at 53 clinical sites

Population: Athletic training students (ATSs) in professional health care education programs

Intervention: E*Value software for tracking patient encounters (PEs); students were asked 3 additional questions upon entering each PE:

1. Did you interact with another athletic trainer (besides the preceptor) during the PE?
2. Did you interact with another health care professional outside of athletic training during the PE?
3. Did you interact with another learner from another health care profession during the PE?

Measurement tool: The previously mentioned 3 survey questions added to the E*Value documentation system at 53 clinical sites where students performed clinical rotations

Findings: Students reported interacting with another athletic trainer in 8.2% of PEs, with a health care professional outside of athletic training in 3.9% of PEs, and with a learner from another health care professional education program in 3.6% of PEs. They reported that they did not incorporate IPCP concepts during 87% of PEs (1,147 of 1,319). They reported IPCP more often in the collegiate setting (21.4% of all reported IPCP PEs), most commonly on head and face injuries (29.2% of IPCP PEs). Athletic training students did not appear to be exposed to IPCP during clinical education as facilitated by their preceptor.

IPEC competency: 3, 4

STUDY AUTHORS: Horbar, Rogowski, Plsek et al. (2001)[12]

Sample size (*n*): 10

Population: U.S. neonatal ICUs and staff

Intervention: Self-selected intensive collaborative QI initiatives over 3 years

Measurement tool: QIs

Findings: Significant decreases in morbidity for critically ill preterm infants; rates were compared with 66 prospectively chosen nonparticipating units.

IPEC competency: 3, 4

STUDY AUTHORS: Kent and Keating (2013)[80]

Sample size (*n*): 18

Population: Undergraduate students in nursing, medicine, PT, OT, social work, and dietetics

Intervention: IP needs assessments twice a week for 8 weeks

Measurement tool: Patient satisfaction survey, postintervention only

Findings: Patients were satisfied with time spent in consultation and collaborative decision making; 94% of patients reported a positive change in their ability to manage self-health issues.

IPEC competency: 3

STUDY AUTHORS: Ketola, Sipila, Makela et al. (2000)[107]

Sample size (*n*): 1,040

Population: Staff from 2 suburban municipal health care centers in Helsinki

Intervention: Intervention group (*n* = 1,040) experienced lectures and meetings of multiprofessional teams, development of local guidelines, and introduction of a structured risk-factor recording sheet as part of patient records from 1995 to 1996; control group with patient records from 1995 (*n* = 1,066) and 1996 (*n* = 1,042)

Measurement tool: QIs

Findings: Intervention group showed improved practice recording cardiovascular risk factors as compared with control patient charts (4a).

IPEC competency: 3

STUDY AUTHORS: Morin, Desrosiers and Gaboury (2018)[108]

Sample size (*n*): 571

Population: Physicians and osteopaths involved with pediatric patients in primary care in Quebec

Intervention: Survey of current practices, attitudes, and barriers regarding IPCP

Measurement tool: Measures of enablers, barriers, and the development of IPCP; structured interviews from a subsample (*n* = 21)

Findings: Personal consultation, professional relationship, and perceived utility of osteopathy and community practice were positively correlated with osteopathic referrals; the strongest predictor was positive clinical results reported by parents. Barriers and enablers were reported.

IPEC competency: 2, 4

STUDY AUTHORS: Zorek, Blaszczyk, Haase, and Raehl (2014)[89]

Sample size (*n*): 20

Population: Pharmacy clinical practice-site preceptors from geriatric and pediatric specializations

Intervention: Qualitative interview to assess readiness of the clinical practice site to facilitate IPCP

Measurement tool: Practice Site Readiness for Interprofessional Education (PRIPE) instrument

Findings: All practice sites were found to train other health care learners (outside of pharmacy). Journal clubs were mentioned as a way to foster IPE during clinical education. Over 50% of preceptors reported meeting the IPEC core competencies related to roles and responsibilities, communication, and teamwork; 80% of preceptors reported their practice (and practice site) fit the definition of *interprofessional*. PRIPE is a useful tool to screen for IPE-ready clinical sites.

IPEC competency: 2, 3, 4

STUDY AUTHORS: Reeves and Freeth (2002)[154]

Sample size (n): 36 students; 38 patients

Population: Orthopedic and rheumatology ward with 27 beds, of which 12 beds were used for the pilot; undergraduate student teams in nursing, medicine, PT, and OT

Intervention: Over 4 weeks, 6 teams (each consisting of 2 students from nursing, 2 from medicine, 1 from OT, and 1 from PT) undertaking the planning and delivery of care (under supervision) for orthopedic and rheumatology patients

Measurement tool: Patient satisfaction survey; data collection from all participants, including students, facilitators, and patients

Findings: Students generally felt that working together in a ward-based team was advantageous for enhancing their teamwork skills; colocating offered immediate interaction with other members of the team. Facilitators struggled to provide effective feedback and found the supervision stressful. They engaged in a 2-day training for the facilitation role. Patients were very satisfied with the care they received and felt they were given more attention; they felt that the students communicated better with them in terms of listening to them, answering their questions, and providing them with the information they needed.

IPEC competency: 3, 4

STUDY AUTHORS: Shafer, Tebb, Pantell et al. (2002)[109]

Sample size (n): 7,920

Population: A total of 10 pediatric clinics in the Kaiser Permanente of Northern California health maintenance organization (HMO)

Intervention: Random assignment of 5 clinics to provide usual care and 5 to provide the intervention, requiring leadership to be engaged by showing the gap between best practice and current practice, a team to be assembled to champion the project, barriers to be identified and solutions developed through monthly meetings, and progress to be monitored with site-specific screening proportions

Measurement tool: QIs

Findings: Of the 1,017 patients eligible for screening in the intervention clinic, 478 (47%) were screened; of 1,194 eligible for screening in the control clinic, 203 (17%) were screened. At baseline, the proportion screened was 0.05 (95% confidence interval [CI], 0.00-0.17) in the intervention and 0.14 (95% CI, 0.01-0.26) in the control clinics. By months 16 to 18, screening rates were 0.65 (95% CI, 0.53-0.77) in the intervention and 0.21 (95% CI, 0.09-0.33) in the control clinics ($F(6, 60) = 5.33$; $P < .001$).

IPEC competency: 3, 4

STUDY AUTHORS: Shirey, White-Williams, Hites et al. (2019)[110]

Sample size (n): 8

Population: IPCP health teams from 7 disciplines at an academic health center in the southeastern United States (nursing, medicine, public health, social work, health services administration, information technology, and other health professions); teams had 8 direct caregivers, consisted of a representative of each discipline, and were augmented with nonlicensed health professionals and community health workers

Intervention: Over a 3-year horizon, targeted strategies for building a high-performing IPCP team based on authentic leadership dimensions; team provided health care to over 250 patients with chronic heart failure, with an emphasis on transitional care services

Measurement tool: Collaborative Practice Assessment Tool (CPAT) using a 7-point Likert scale

Findings: Evolution of the team ranged as follows: communication and information exchange (4.0-6.8), decision making and conflict management (2.3-7.0), and patient involvement in team care (5.7-7.0).

IPEC competency: 3, 4

STUDY AUTHORS: Shiyanbola, Randall, Lammers et al. (2014)[70]

Sample size (*n*): 30

Population: Undergraduate students in nursing, medicine, pharmacy, dental hygiene, and nutrition

Intervention: Student-led diabetes self-management and health promotion education program for underserved patients; 6-month longitudinal program

Measurement tool: Pre- and posttest comparison of knowledge (student and patient) and clinical lab tests; patient satisfaction survey

Findings: Significant improvements were shown in patients' diabetes knowledge, diabetes management, and improvement in clinical outcomes. Significant improvements were also shown in the students' ability to educate patients about diabetes management and in their awareness of team care roles in diabetes cases.

IPEC competency: 3

STUDY AUTHORS: Magnan, Solberg, Kottke et al. (1998)[111]

Sample size (*n*): Unknown

Population: A total of 44 primary care clinics (contracting with 2 large managed care organizations [MCOs]) randomized to a comparison (C) or an intervention (I) group

Intervention: Training plus ongoing consultation and networking for clinic team leaders in the intervention group

Measurement tool: CQIs

Findings: All 22 (I) clinics identified teams that appeared to follow the 7-step improvement process. The mean numbers of system processes were identical at baseline, 11.2 (I) versus 12.1 (C). After the intervention, this had changed to 25.8 (I) clinics versus 11.3 (C) clinics ($P = .022$).

IPEC competency: 3, 4

STUDY AUTHORS: van Eeghen, Littenberg, and Kessler (2018)[155]

Sample size (*n*): 10

Population: Type 2 diabetic patients ($n = 10$); control group ($n = 106$)

Intervention: Implementation of a pilot stepped-care model including a community health nurse and workflow redesign to include behavioral health services

Measurement tool: Patient hemoglobin A1C (HbA1C) results; days between HbA1C tests

Findings: Compared with the control group, patient outcomes improved for both test results and process of reporting for tests (measured by time between tests); differences were not significant.

IPEC competency: 3, 4

Influence of Online Delivery Models on Attitudes and IPCP

Educational strategies for the delivery of IPE varied within the literature. A trend exists in education that shifts content delivery from a traditional classroom where students and instructors meet face to face to a delivery format that is either partially online (blended) or online at a distance.[46] IPE has been employed in all 3 of these configurations as instructional delivery options.

McKee, D'Eon, and Trinder[47] determined that before students can engage in problem solving during IPE activities, they must have knowledge and information. With a trend toward online activities, a blended learning environment is a natural progression for the delivery of IPE activities.

The use of technology to promote learning has been increasing in the education of health professionals.[48] Supplementing the traditional classroom with an online component is considered a blended learning environment. IPE has also been delivered in this manner. The use of technology in **blended IPE** activities was meant to overcome some of the barriers inherent in IPE.[49] Chen and colleagues[49] identified that students rated the obtaining of learning objectives as high in this environment; however, they valued the face-to-face component more than the online component.

The use of alternative technological methodologies (e.g., online simulation, asynchronous case discussion) had positive implications for student attitudes toward health care teams and IPCP.[31] The use of technology-driven communication methodologies in IPCP has also been found to improve access and contact with care providers and reduce waiting periods between team members.[50] It was also shown that, although this enhanced ability to communicate through technology offers advantages, it can also create interruptions in a provider's day due to increased accessibility. Regardless of the pros and cons, technology is increasingly infused into IPCP practice, and thus the importance of technology-driven IPE experiences cannot be ignored.[98] Schack-Dugré[98] concluded that with the expansion of global health initiatives, telehealth, and medical tourism, the necessity for team collaboration within an online or electronic format is on the rise. The ideal format for educating the health care team across geographic or health system borders is through online IPE.

There have been numerous approaches to the delivery of IPE: group problem solving, seminar-based discussions, role-playing, or any combination of these.[51] Within these broad categories are also differences in **synchronous** versus **asynchronous activities**. Success in meeting learning objectives depends on the instructional model used to foster the IPE experience. Additionally, research is needed to better understand which delivery models optimize the IPE experience.[51]

As stated, communication in a distance environment can be synchronous or asynchronous. Synchronous interaction occurs when students interact simultaneously with each other or faculty; feedback and facilitation are provided instantaneously.[52] An example of synchronous communication in distance education would be a web conference or a live chat. Video may or may not be used. McCutcheon and colleagues[51] found that the use of video in several studies provided an environment for students to observe other professions in action when compared with reading or talking, and this led to higher trust between health professionals. The use of virtual environments increased interprofessional socialization and was thought to translate to improved capacity for teamwork.[51] The virtual environment allowed the participants to work together and visualize their recommendations for a greater patient-centered experience.

Effectiveness of Simulation

Simulation activities are frequently used in IPE to authenticate and reinforce learning.[57,58] A systematic review conducted by Ryall, Judd, and Gordon[59] found that simulation activities for engaging and assessing learners are becoming ubiquitous in health professions education. Simulation can also mitigate the barriers of insufficient accessibility of clinical site placements and safety concerns for students who are working toward achieving competency while involved in direct patient care.[60-62] Simulations have been widely studied and proven to provide a safe environment for repetitive deliberate practice. Additionally, simulation is a learner-centered experience, whereas in clinical practice settings, learning occurs in a patient-centered environment.[63]

Evans and colleagues[64] studied the effects of a fully online IPE course using both synchronous and asynchronous interaction strategies. The study revealed that entry-level students' perceptions of interprofessional interactions and relationships were positive. Additionally, increased confidence in other health professionals' roles was noted. However, changes were insignificant regarding perceptions of their communication and teamwork skills following completion of the course. Student attitudes toward IPE were not significantly changed postintervention; however, it is worth noting that students already had a positive attitude toward interprofessional relationships prior to the intervention (Evans et al., 2014).[64]

Assessment Tools

Assessing the effectiveness of IPE is challenging; no measure has yet to be broadly accepted or adopted.[71-73] Although NCIPE provides a repository of tools equipped with psychometrics and evidence of recent use, researchers fail to convene on a set of tools to assess IPE and IPCP. Table 4.5 displays the most commonly used assessment tools for IPE and IPCP across contemporary literature, categorized by Kirkpatrick's expanded outcomes typology. Additionally, the studies providing the psychometric data (validity and reliability), as well as the IPEC competency domain, are included to guide researchers to the best tool.

The IPEC core competency domains were introduced in chapter 1 and surface again here as essential elements of IPE program assessment. The core competency domains are as follows[53]:

- Values and ethics
- Roles and responsibilities
- Interprofessional communication
- Teams and teamwork

Table 4.5 Interprofessional Assessment Tools

Level of Evaluation	Tool	Description	Subscales	Psychometrics	IPEC Core Competencies
1	Readiness for Interprofessional Learning Scale (RIPLS)	19-item tool designed to measure readiness of students for IPE	1. Teamwork and collaboration 2. Professional identity 3. Roles and responsibilities	Parsell and Bligh (1999)[117]	1, 2, 3, 4
1, 2a	Interdisciplinary Education Perception Scale (IEPS)	18-item survey measuring the impact of interprofessional experiences on health care students	1. Competence and autonomy 2. Perceived need for cooperation 3. Perception of actual cooperation 4. 4. Understanding of others' values	Hawk, Buckwalter, Byrd et al. (2002)[118]	1, 2, 4
2a	Attitudes Toward Health Care Teams Scale (ATHCTS-R)	14-item instrument assessing the attitudes of students learning about team care	1. Quality of care 2. Time constraints	Heinemann, Schmitt, Farrell et al. (1999);[119] Curran, Sharpe, Forristall et al. (2007)[120]	2
2a	Entry-Level Interprofessional Questionnaire (ELIQ)	27-item questionnaire measuring student attitudes toward IPE and collaboration	1. Communication and teamwork 2. Interprofessional learning 3. Interprofessional interaction 4. Perceptions of relationships with colleagues	Pollard, Miers, and Gilchrist (2005)[56]	1
1, 2b	TeamSTEPPS Teamwork Attitudes Questionnaire (T-TAQ)	30-item questionnaire assessing the impact of IPE on health professionals' knowledge, attitudes, and team skills	1. Team structure 2. Leadership 3. Situation management 4. Mutual support 5. Communication	Baker, Krokos, and Amodeo (2008)[116]	3, 4
2a	Student Perceptions of Interprofessional Clinical Education Revised, Version 2 (SPICE-R2)	10-item self-assessment measuring students' perceptions of IPE and IPCP	1. Interprofessional teamwork and team-based practice 2. Roles and responsibilities for collaborative practice 3. Patient outcomes from collaborative practice	Zorek, Fike, Eickhoff et al. (2016)[121]	1, 2, 4

Level of Evaluation	Tool	Description	Subscales	Psychometrics	IPEC Core Competencies
3, 4a	Interprofessional Socialization and Valuing Scale (ISVS-21)	21-item self-report instrument measuring interprofessional socialization among students and health practitioners and their readiness to function on interprofessional teams	1. Beliefs 2. Attitudes 3. Behaviors	King, Orchard, Khalili et al. (2016)[122]	1, 2, 3, 4
3	Assessment of Interprofessional Team Collaboration Scale (AITCS)	37-item self-report instrument evaluating IPCP among a variety of health care teams	1. Partnership 2. Cooperation 3. Coordination	Orchard, King, Khalili et al. (2012)[123]	4
3	Team Skills Scale (TSS)	17-item self-assessment of skills required to collaborate effectively on a geriatric care team	1. Interpersonal skills 2. Discipline-specific skills 3. Geriatric care skills 4. Team skills	Grymonpre, van Ineveld, Nelson et al. (2010)[124]	2, 3, 4
3	Interprofessional Collaborator Assessment Rubric (ICAR)	31-item observer tool using rubric scoring to assess learners' achievement of interprofessional competency domains; learners may need to be assessed multiple times for maximum reliability	1. Communication 2. Collaboration 3. Roles and responsibilities 4. Collaborative patient-centered approach 5. Team functioning	Curran, Hollett, Casimiro et al. (2011)[125]	1, 3, 4
3	Interprofessional Collaborative Competency Attainment Survey (ICCAS)	20-item self-assessment of the Canadian competencies of interprofessional care	None	Archibold, Trumpower, and MacDonald (2014)[126]	1, 2, 3, 4
3	Interprofessional Collaboration Scale (ICS)	13-item round-robin observer assessment tool measuring IPCP of target groups	1. Communication 2. Accommodation 3. Isolation	Kenaszchuk, Reeves, Nicholas et al. (2010)[127]	1, 3, 4

(continued)

Table 4.5 *(continued)*

Level of Evaluation	Tool	Description	Subscales	Psychometrics	IPEC Core Competencies
3	IPEC Competency Survey	42-item self-assessment of achievement of the IPEC competencies	1. Ethics and values 2. Roles and responsibilities 3. Interprofessional communication 4. Teams and teamwork	Dow, DiasGrandos, Mazmanian et al. (2014)[128]	1, 2, 3, 4
3	Interdisciplinary Team Performance Scale (ITPS)	59-item self-assessment of interprofessional team performance in long-term care	1. Leadership 2. Communication 3. Coordination 4. Conflict management 5. Team cohesion 6. Perceived unit effectiveness	Temkin-Greener, Gross, Kunitz et al. (2004)[129]	4
3	Observed Interprofessional Collaboration (OIPC)	20-item observer tool assessing interprofessional behaviors during team meetings	1. Purpose of meeting 2. Team composition 3. Expertise affirmation 4. Attainment of consensus 5. Person-centered practice 6. Communication 7. Respectful attitude 8. Facilitation and mediation 9. Shared decision making 10. Adoption of shared plan	Careau, Vincent, Swaine et al. (2014)[130]	3, 4
3	Performance Assessment for Communication and Teamwork (PACT)	13-item observer tool assessing communication and teamwork during simulation	1. Team structure 2. Leadership 3. Situation monitoring 4. Mutual support 5. Communication	Chiu (2014)[131]	2
4a	Index of Interdisciplinary Collaboration (IIC)	42-item survey measuring aspects and levels of IPCP within an organization	1. Interdependence and flexibility 2. Newly created professional activities 3. Collective ownership of goal 4. Reflection on process	Parker Oliver, Wittenberg-Lyles, and Day (2007)[132]	1
4a	Healthcare Team Vitality Instrument (HTVI)	10-item tool assessing health care team functioning; QIs and innovative initiatives	1. Support structures 2. Engagement and empowerment 3. Patient care transitions 4. Team communication	Upenieks, Lee, Flanagan et al. (2010)[133]	2, 3, 4

The 2016 update to the core competencies can be found through an Internet search using the key term "2016 IPEC IPE core competencies." Health professions programs often center their IPE efforts across the 4 competency domains, preparing their students with the knowledge and skills necessary to function on and lead interprofessional care teams. Table 4.6 connects the dots between the IPEC competencies and Kirkpatrick's levels of evaluation by outlining potential tools for use in IPE assessment. Each tool is accompanied by a scenario or implementation example, making selection easer for the novice researcher or IPE program administrator.

Table 4.6 Examples of Assessment by IPEC Domain

Level of Evaluation	Tool	Implementation Example	IPEC Competencies Assessed
1	Readiness for Interprofessional Learning Scale (RIPLS)	Gathering of baseline data at the beginning of a program; comparison of students across health care professions	1, 2, 3, 4
2a	Interdisciplinary Education Perception Scale (IEPS)	Pre- and posttest alongside an IPE simulation; combine with tool that measures communication	1, 2, 4
2b	TeamSTEPPS Teamwork Attitudes Questionnaire (T-TAQ)	Pre- and posttest alongside a TeamSTEPPS workshop	3, 4
3	Interprofessional Socialization and Valuing Scale (ISVS-21)	Pre- and posttest around set of IPE modules in an online course	1, 2, 3, 4
4a	Healthcare Team Vitality Instrument (HTVI)	Team assessment before and after innovative patient care initiative	2, 3, 4

Summary

This chapter covered the current literature on IPE and IPCP using Kirkpatrick's expanded outcomes typology as an organizational framework. Each section of the review synthesized the findings related to Kirkpatrick's typology and identified gaps in the body of evidence. Additionally, the reader is now able to apply evidence related to IPE and IPCP in the classroom and practice setting and use assessment strategies and tools appropriate for the planned level of assessment.

The evidence of practice and system change is new and growing in strength and depth, and it has painted a landscape of hope, of promise for the future of health care delivery. Furthermore, the evidence is shifting to align with the Triple and Quadruple Aims, highlighting the impact of IPE and IPCP on practice behaviors[56, 70, 74-77] and clinical outcomes.[78-80] It is evident that organizations, accreditors, faculty members, and students see the value in IPE and IPCP, resulting in more programs generating more evidence to support their effectiveness. Although this chapter showcased research to date that is overwhelmingly positive, taking a mindful approach to IPE and IPCP is warranted. Creating a robust, accessible curriculum and planning authentic, impactful team collaborations is challenging and often requires institutional support.

Questions remain regarding the impact of IPE on student preparedness. Environmental factors challenge the replication of evidence across settings, creating a database of single-study findings, which are not as powerful as a series of corroborated conclusions. Lockeman and colleagues[11] found that a greater rigor of assessment strategies in IPE activities coupled with the use of a triangulated measurement strategy will provide data to guide decision making on IPE development until more research has been completed. Additionally, the partnering of educators with health delivery organizations where actual practice occurs is deficient; attempts to align and implement education opportunities are infrequently assimilated well within health systems, lending challenges to implementation and examination for efficacy.

Furthermore, a systematic review of IPE program effectiveness and associated outcomes uncovered that IPE could not be generalized easily; however, the trend toward improved implementation of IPE around the world was noted to be continuously occurring.[30] Complicating assessment and generalization, the range of approaches for delivering IPE, the lack of standardized competencies within professional programs and between disciplines, and the diverse set of assessment tools are contributing factors for the scarcity of scientific evidence.[81]

Faculty champions and leaders of interprofessional teams in practice settings must continue to move the needle by striving to improve patient care through interprofessional teaming and assessment of programs and initiatives to fill the gaps in the literature and strengthen the evidence. NAM reached the following conclusions and made the following recommendations through the Committee on Measuring the Impact of IPE on Collaborative Practice and Patient Outcomes[29]:

1. Align the education and health care delivery systems more closely.
2. Develop a conceptual framework for measuring the impact of IPE.
3. Strengthen the evidence base for IPE.
4. Link IPE with changes in collaborative behavior.

- *Conclusion 1*—Without a purposeful and more comprehensive system of engagement between the education and health care delivery systems, evaluating the impact of IPE interventions on health and system outcomes will be difficult.
- *Conclusion 2*—Having a comprehensive conceptual model would greatly enhance the description and purpose of IPE interventions and their potential impact. Such a model would provide a consistent taxonomy and framework for strengthening the evidence base linking IPE with health and system outcomes.
- *Conclusion 3*—More purposeful, well-designed, and thoughtfully reported studies are needed to answer key questions about the effectiveness of IPE in improving performance in practice and health and system outcomes.

- *Recommendation 1*—Interprofessional stakeholders, funders, and policy makers should commit resources to a coordinated series of well-designed studies of the association between IPE and collaborative behavior, including teamwork and performance in practice. These studies should focus on developing broad consensus on how to measure IPCP effectively across a range of learning environments, patient populations, and practice settings.

- *Recommendation 2*—Educators and academic and health system leaders should adopt a mixed-methods research approach for evaluating the impact of IPE on health and system outcomes. When possible, such studies should include an economic analysis and be carried out by teams of experts that include educational evaluators, health services researchers, and economists, along with educators and others engaged in IPE.

Chapters 5 through 7 will transition from a focus on IPE to an in-depth review of IPCP. The next chapter will expand upon the importance of the relationship between health care professionals, including the value of shared goals, and improvement in quality as an outcome of engaged teams.

CASE STUDY Debriefing

Though the faculty voted to segregate the students from the two professions, MPE was occurring in this case, which is not the same as IPE. While PT and OT students shared the classroom and were led by members of the profession they aspired to join, they were not learning about each other or from each other as students; they were learning with each other only. Additionally, it appears that a perceived hierarchy swayed the vote or differentiated roles in patient care. This, combined with a lack of respect for IPE and for peer professions in health care, violates the premise of the IPEC competencies. These include values and ethics related to IPCP, understanding of roles and responsibilities, interprofessional communication, and team and teamwork skills.[53] Effective change begins with professional development of the faculty who will lead the IPE initiative (see chapter 3 for examples).

Case Study Discussion Questions

1. Consider ways for June to be a change agent in her educational setting. Based on the case presented, what are her main targets, and how might she begin her quest?
2. June's colleague presented professional role stereotypes as a rationale for segregating the health care classroom. How does his belief affect IPE at June's school? Which IPEC competency does this relate to, and how might June respond to him?
3. Barriers to IPE are commonly mentioned as reasons for not advancing IPE efforts. What are the barriers apparent in this case? Present them connected to Kirkpatrick's typology, and propose potential solutions.

CHAPTER 5

Building or Rebuilding Interprofessional Relationships

K. Michelle Knewstep-Watkins, OTD, OTR/L
C. Michelle Longley, MSN, RN, NP-C
Meghan M. Scanlon, BSIE

Objectives

After reading this chapter, the reader will be able to do the following:

- Identify the value of a shared goal for building an interprofessional care team.
- Describe the importance of engaging frontline health care providers and members who can provide knowledge and diversity to a care team.
- Identify strategies to construct an interprofessional team.
- Describe common stages of team development.
- Identify team assessment tools and QI (quality improvement) methodologies that facilitate IPCP.

CASE STUDY Interprofessional Fall Prevention Program

Christine, an advanced practice nurse, has been leading the fall prevention program in her academic medical center for nearly 5 years. Although the organization has experienced fewer falls than many peer organizations, falls continue to occur. The Fall Champion Team of nurses has inconsistent attendance at monthly meetings, and members report that no one on their units pays attention to their education or recommendations because everyone is too busy to do more. Though rates of falls with injuries are not increasing, this conventional approach is not yielding any significant or sustained reduction in total falls or falls with injuries. To renew the focus on fall prevention, an internationally renowned expert is consulted, and

(continued)

Case Study *(continued)*

after a thorough on-site evaluation, she recommends adoption of a multifactorial, interprofessional fall prevention program.

With executive leadership support, Christine invites Kevin, an engaged, enthusiastic OT, to colead the fall prevention program, and the two interprofessional leads agree to reorganize the entire program structure. Kevin's academic OT program incorporated IPE each semester, so he is accustomed to working closely with nurses, physicians, social workers, SLPs, PTs, and other team members. After graduating and joining the 650-bed academic medical center where Christine works, he has experienced clinical practice and patient care performed with limited integration and communication between all members of the team. This functional structure of work is often known as work in silos.

After Kevin accepts Christine's invitation to share the leadership role in the fall prevention program, he finds himself surrounded by nurses who are apprehensive of his leadership in their historically nurse-driven safety program. Likewise, Kevin is hesitant to volunteer suggestions or ideas due to feeling like an outsider. This bidirectional hesitancy impedes effective communication and therefore effective collaboration and teamwork.

Shortly after the start of their partnership, Kevin and Christine's organization gains a high-level leader who brings Lean methodology to the medical center (see the Lean Methodology section later in this chapter for more information). Setting a True North goal to "be the safest place to receive and provide care," Kevin and Christine have a renewed prioritization of fall injury prevention. Under the guidance of Marie, a Lean expert, Christine and Kevin perform a brief gap analysis and immediately expand the frontline clinician Fall Champion Team to include OTs, PTs, patient sitters, transportation providers, phlebotomists, radiology technologists, patient care assistants (PCAs), central equipment room staff, float-pool clinicians, and an ad hoc administrator. Based on feedback from existing and new members, the meeting schedule and location are modified to accommodate everyone's schedules, and conference calling is made available for those unable to attend in person. Attendance expands from 2 to 3 participants each month to 20 to 25 participants every other week. With a clear organizational goal, systemic QI methodology, and consistent clinician participation, the new interprofessional Fall Champions are poised to transform the fall prevention program.

The interprofessional Fall Champions identify fall prevention vulnerabilities using the A3 tool for system-level fall challenges and brainstorm interprofessional strategies to improve patient safety. Using organizational data on fall events, Christine, Kevin, and the Fall Champions focus on improving safety related to mobilizing and toileting high-risk patients with coaching and mentoring from Marie. Their A3 focuses on falls in which patients are assisted to the floor by clinicians. From frontline clinician feedback, the team learns that members do not consistently know how to safely ambulate a patient. A communication tool, the Out-of-Bed Plan, is developed with interprofessional feedback and is tested on 4 units. This communication tool is a laminated sign that allows clinicians to circle what assistive devices a patient needs to mobilize (e.g., cane, walker, crutches, gait belt) and the safest method of toileting (e.g., bedpan, bedside commode, toilet).

After positive clinician feedback and consistent daily compliance filling out the Out-of-Bed Plan on the test units, the laminated signs are distributed to all units across the organization. Clinician feedback and daily compliance continue to be monitored for education or supply needs for the next 6 months. During that time, assisted falls during ambulation and toileting decrease by 78%, and falls with injury during ambulation decrease by 90%. After 2 years of using the Out-of-Bed Plan, the organization installs templated dry-erase boards in all patient rooms to communicate patient needs and include all elements of the Out-of-Bed mobility and toileting safety components.

According to NAM (formerly IOM) and the Joint Commission, most medical errors are related to miscommunication, and improving interprofessional collaboration is vital to reducing the majority of medical errors.[1] Thus, the role and impact of IPCP in health care, as well as the educational efforts to facilitate it, have been gaining attention in recent decades, as shown by the increasing visibility and volume in literature.[2-4] The complexity of health care is increased by the broad spectrum of levels of patient acuity as well as the extensive diversity of health care team members, including professions, level of experience, education, and professionalism. This presents an enigmatic challenge to clarifying best practices in education, training, and providing care. Trends in literature assert that deficits in teamwork and communication contribute to problems in safe, appropriate patient care.[2,4] This chapter will share content on understanding, creating, and fostering teamwork to support IPCP.

A unique feature of the health care team serving patients is that this team is composed of varying types of direct and indirect health care employees. **Direct health care providers** include providers who directly interact with the patient, such as a bedside nurse. **Indirect health care providers** perform services that support direct care providers, such as a nurse who works in health informatics. The health care team experiences evolution temporally, which includes the influence of new clinicians arriving, clinicians resigning, and clinicians taking on new roles. A team in health care can come in many sizes; it could include the individuals who work on a cardiac unit in the medical center, or it could consist of the individuals who function as a work group to address a safety initiative, such as reducing patient falls in a medical center. Often, QI or program development efforts in health care are addressed by a group of individuals who represent a larger group of employees. In all these cases, there is a group of individual employees whose efforts and services can be improved through teamwork.

There are known strategies and tools for facilitating focused, effective IPCP in health care. These include methods for developing attributes that promote effective interpersonal relationships and communication, sometimes referred to as **soft skills**, as well as strategies and tools to facilitate focused group efforts. The chapter will address methods to promote productive collaboration in order to identify goals for improvement and how to approach these goals as a strategic health care team.

Evidence and Current Practice

A significant proportion of the current literature on interprofessionalism focuses on education at the undergraduate and graduate levels. This foundational IPE model is essential for new clinicians, as highlighted by NAM:

> Inadequate preparation of health professionals for working together, especially in interprofessional teams, has been implicated in a range of adverse outcomes, including lower provider and patient satisfaction, greater number of medical errors and other patient safety issues, low workforce retention, system inefficiencies resulting in higher costs, and suboptimal community engagement.[3(p12)]

A systematic review revealed that 78% of studies reported positive outcomes when organizational practice changes (Kirkpatrick's level 4a) were measured as an outcome of IPE.[5,6] Similarly, another study found multidimensional gains in their systematic review and meta-analysis of IPE related to team members' job satisfaction (Quadruple Aim; see chapter 4), caring for complex patient needs (Kirkpatrick's level 4b), and interprofessional collaboration (Kirkpatrick's level 3).[7]

As defined by WHO, interprofessional practice involves "multiple health workers from different professional backgrounds working together with patients, families, caregivers, and communities to deliver the highest quality of care."[8(p7)] In addition to an emphasis on IPE, current literature that focuses on interprofessional collaboration concentrates on highly specific patient populations or includes limited inclusion of relevant professions beyond physicians and nurses. Thus, there are opportunities for future research and literature to explore interprofessional collaboration across varying patient populations as well as among a variety of health care providers. This gap in existing literature on the translation of IPE and IPCP beyond formal graduate and undergraduate programs and across populations and disciplines implies systematic vulnerabilities in existing health care structures.

Additionally, when new graduates enter the health care arena armed with interprofessional skills and expectations from formal academia, collaborative methodologies may not always be fostered, encouraged, or even well received by the veteran health care providers. Organizations must prioritize a culture in which interprofessional care providers acquire the KSAs (knowledge, skills, and attitudes) to practice collaboratively through education, training, and interprofessional health care team development.[9]

Interprofessional Team Composition

Creating a highly effective health care team is rarely as simple as assembling a group of providers who are knowledgeable and experienced in their clinical practice. Commonly, the group members who will become a health care team are diverse with regard to knowledge, experience, values, and expectations. These differences can present challenges in aligning the team toward a common purpose and accepted processes for meeting the goals.

In some cases, there is an established group of experienced health care providers who have been working together to meet patient needs. These providers may have worked this way for decades, shared many experiences, developed their professional identities in relation to one another, and developed long-standing meaningful friendships. It is critical to recognize that the group may be diverse in the number of years of experience and years working together, which can mean there are established roles, routines, and habits well beyond the simple norms of a scope of practice. However, this does not necessarily mean that these health care providers are a high-functioning team. Similarly, other groups may have a majority of entry-level providers or providers who are new to the group or to serving a particular population, but these characteristics do not necessarily imply that they are a poorly functioning team.

A health care team is effective when all team members understand their role as part of the team as well as the roles and areas of expertise of other team members. One's role on a health care team should not be dictated wholly by profession. For example, patient safety is not solely the responsibility or role of nurses; instead, it is recognized as a shared role. However, it is important to recognize the recommendation of a dietitian in the creation of a patient's nutritional intake, because the dietitian is the professional with the greatest content knowledge in this area, even if other providers have an understanding of nutrition. See chapter 4 for a review of the evidence highlighting the impact of years of experience on IPE and IPCP.

Collaborative workplace environments are routinely associated with improved patient outcomes due to effective workflows and synergistic relationships. Even with shared goals and collaborative relationships, such environments require intentionality. Conflict is an inevitable part of working in teams and stems from individual, contextual, and intrapersonal characteristics that can significantly impair team cohesion and objectives.[10] It is important for team participants and leaders to be familiar with sources of group conflict and implement strategies to resolve conflict effectively.

COLLABORATIVE CORNER
Sources of Conflict

Conflict can arise from individual characteristics, contextual factors, or intrapersonal conditions.[11]

- *Individual characteristics*—Individual team members enter group settings from different backgrounds with individualized values, opinions, and experiences that lead to assumptions about patient care needs and how to meet them.

- *Contextual factors*—Situations in which roles and responsibilities are unclear or group goals lack clarity can cause stress and conflict, particularly when combined with fast-paced environments, unpredictability, or high-stakes outcomes.

- *Intrapersonal conditions*—Conflict is common in circumstances of actual or perceived hierarchical relationships, inconsistent team membership and participation, or limited member or group accountability.

What methods or activities might assist in identifying and addressing individual characteristics, contextual factors, and intrapersonal conditions that contribute to conflict?

EBP OF TEAMSHIP
The Relationship Between Patient Safety and Team Behaviors

Layne and colleagues completed a descriptive correlational study to investigate the relationships between negative behaviors of health care employees and perceptions of patient safety culture. This study was conducted in the acute care environments of a health system that included an academic medical center and affiliated community hospitals. Study participants were direct care providers as well as support service providers, and participants engaged in the study anonymously through an online survey. The study used the Negative Behaviors in HealthCare survey (NBHC) and the Hospital Survey on Patient Safety Culture (HSOPS) to investigate these relationships.

The researchers highlight several meaningful correlations from the study. There was a relationship of increased level of teamwork, management support for patient safety, and openness of communication in health care units with less exposure to contributing factors of negative behaviors among health care employees. Participants who reported a higher fear of retaliation demonstrated a correlation with a lower overall patient safety grade.

Layne and colleagues advocate for further investigation in this area for a greater understanding of teamwork for patient care as well as for understanding job satisfaction of health care providers.[23]

It is also valuable to recognize that teaming in a health care organization occurs on many levels. A *team* is defined as a group of people who assemble to achieve a common goal, which can occur in any organization regardless of size or complexity. Thus, health care organizations are composed of many layers of teams. The organization as a whole is a team, and additional levels of health care teams are nested within the organization to address cascading goals of the central goal. A medical center may also have diagnosis-centered service areas, such as orthopedics, which are teams within the organization. Additionally, formal teams can assemble to meet a specific need, such as a patient education committee, or informal teams may emerge organically in order to collaborate and address a concern.

Health Care Organization Appraisal

The earliest stage of developing a highly effective health care team is for the people in leadership to thoughtfully and respectfully appraise the effectiveness of the current group or organization. Simply put, this is when leaders identify problem areas and opportunities for improvement. The depth and breadth of the appraisal phase depend on the size and complexity of the organization. A small medical practice and a large health system both need an appraisal of current workflow and work groups. However, the complexity of the appraisal will directly correlate with the complexity of the organization.

The appraisal is not a judgmental review. It cannot be an assessment of who is better or worse at their role, nor should it be about which roles are the most valuable or important. The general points of appraisal are as follows:

- What are the most meaningful areas for improvement in the health care provided by this organization? What metrics or deficits in patient care need improvement?

- What are this organization's strategic goals regarding the areas that need improvement?

- For larger organizations, what change management tools should be used to more extensively assess the current status? Change management tools include stakeholder analysis, stakeholder expectations, and business needs assessment.

- How have these areas for improvement been measured previously? Further, how should success in the strategic goals be measured using both qualitative and quantitative measures?

- Who are the direct and indirect care providers involved in this work? How do these professions influence the group?

- Are all professions, including both direct and indirect providers, engaged in the flow of dialogue and included in the regular meetings?

- What is the plan for effective communication? What groups (or audiences) need to be updated or asked for information as part of this process? What method or tool will be used to connect with these groups and at what frequency?

- What behaviors are expected from leaders or other key groups in order to ensure the work progresses?

The people appraising the current state of group functioning typically serve in roles that supervise the group members or are leadership sponsors of the work assigned to the group. These supervisors may have to prepare the organization for upcoming changes to allow for development. The health care providers will likely require time away from their direct care duties in order to participate in the development of the team and associated goals. The supervisors may need to address the staffing levels and staff schedules to ensure that health care responsibilities are being met. They may also recognize that team development initiatives require expertise beyond their own, in which case they may hire external consultants to help with observing current workflow dynamics and implementing the initial meetings.

Value of a Meaningful, Common Goal

The identification of a central, meaningful, and impactful strategy, or **True North goal**, for the health care agency is the foundation of developing effective health care teams. A critical role of leadership is to establish a goal that sets the direction for where the organization is working to go, speaks to the hearts and minds of the people, and serves to motivate, engage, and inspire the entire organization. This True North goal should reflect the ideal goal or perfect condition to be achieved by the organization, such as to become the best place to receive and provide care. One example of this ideal situation could be that no one, patient or worker, suffers harm in the organization. The True North goals for measures of harm for patients could be zero infections and for workers could be zero injuries. Setting True North

THINKING ABOUT TRUE NORTH

To understand True North, consider the idea of trying to reach the horizon. It appears to be far off in the distance. Looking at it shows directionally which way to go. The steps taken toward it will always be progress in that direction. However, it is a fixed point that seemingly remains a constant distance away even when progress is made toward it. It provides orientation to the direction of travel, motivates and inspires continued progress, and serves as a constant reminder of what everyone is working toward.

goals at perfect helps to focus the organization, demonstrate that the status quo is not acceptable, and unleash the energy of everyone in the organization toward achieving the goals.

Leaders are responsible for setting the True North or direction for the organization, but they cannot simply tell people how to achieve it. The True North cannot be achieved without the alignment and energy of everyone in the organization working together toward the common goal. The organization itself is a team, and good leaders recognize that each individual in the organization is critical to the success of that team. Once the True North has been set by leadership, the work becomes figuring out how the True North goal cascades throughout the organization. As the experts in their domains, all members need to determine how the work they do every day moves the organization toward achieving True North and how they will measure their impact on that goal. This work should happen iteratively throughout the levels of leadership from the frontline or caregivers to the top leaders until goals exist at each level in the organization and are aligned to True North (see figure 5.1). The work of the highest level of leadership is to set the direction or course for the organization through the top-level goals; the work of everyone else is to understand how their work enables the achievement of those goals. The goals should be tied directly to the strategic plan of the organization.

As an organization works to determine cascading goals, note that the type of goal depends on what level in the organization is being measured. Working from True North, the first few levels of goals into the organization will likely be lagging indicators or **outcome measures** that will take a long-term, focused effort to make substantial progress and improvement. Improvement on these types of measures can be slow. Lagging indicators are also typically easy to measure because outcome data are common in electronic systems.

As goals are established through the organization, the areas that are closer to the provision of direct care need to understand more quickly the cause-and-effect relationships between the improvements being made and the impact they have on the problems at hand. The type of measures that are needed at these levels are likely **leading indicators**. Leading indicators are typically **process measures**, which makes them harder to collect from an electronic system and more likely to be gathered through manual data collection. Observation is a great way to collect data on leading indicators, but it can be time consuming. Process measures are commonly

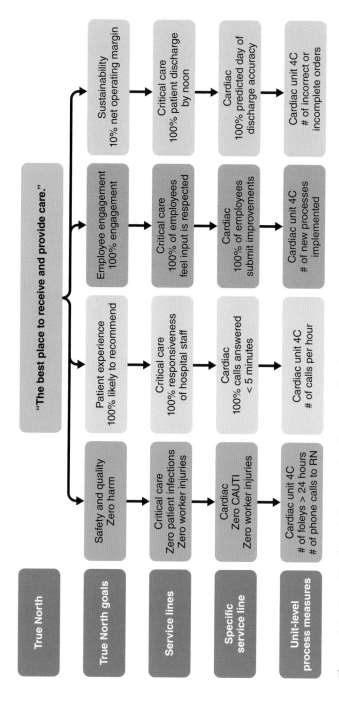

Figure 5.1 True North and the cascade of organizational goals.

True North

"The best place to receive and provide care."

True North goals

| Safety and quality Zero harm | Patient experience 100% likely to recommend | Employee engagement 100% engagement | Sustainability 10% net operating margin |

Service lines

| Critical care Zero patient infections Zero worker injuries | Critical care 100% responsiveness of hospital staff | Critical care 100% of employees feel input is respected | Critical care 100% patient discharge by noon |

Specific service line

| Cardiac Zero CAUTI Zero worker injuries | Cardiac 100% calls answered < 5 minutes | Cardiac 100% of employees submit improvements | Cardiac 100% predicted day of discharge accuracy |

Unit-level process measures

| Cardiac unit 4C # of foleys > 24 hours # of phone calls to RN | Cardiac unit 4C # of calls per hour | Cardiac unit 4C # of new processes implemented | Cardiac unit 4C # of incorrect or incomplete orders |

COLLABORATIVE CORNER
Determining Cascading Organizational Goals

At ABC Health System, leaders had just aligned around the True North of being the best place to receive and provide care. The True North goals were safety and quality, patient experience, employee engagement, and sustainability, and the measures for each goal were set at perfect. Once the leaders finalized the strategy for the organization, they worked to engage their direct reports in the process. Sue, the chief nurse, engaged with Steve, VP of emergency services; Cheryl, VP of critical care services; and Diane, VP of ambulatory care, to ask them what the biggest opportunities were for the service lines in support of zero harm. After discussion as a team and reviewing last year's data, they aligned around zero patient infections and zero worker injuries. They all agreed to work to engage their direct reports in the process.

Cheryl scheduled one-on-one sessions with each of her directors. In Cheryl's discussion with Laura, director of cardiac, they reviewed last year's data and talked about the current improvement initiatives going on in cardiac services. Laura and Cheryl agreed that focusing on eliminating catheter-associated urinary tract infections (CAUTI) was where cardiac services could make the most progress toward the goal of zero infections. From a worker perspective, the idea that one injury was too many still resonated with Laura, so she chose to keep the goal of zero worker injuries to maintain that focus.

Cheryl asked Laura to engage with her units in defining process measures that they could track in as close to real time as possible to show how each unit was working toward zero harm. Laura reached out to her team to schedule one-on-one time for these discussions. In her session with Debbie, nurse manager on 4C, Laura learned that a lot of patients on 4C arrived with catheters, and it was important to make sure they were removed within 48 hours to eliminate the risk of CAUTI. In order to meet the 48-hour goal, she thought if they knew how many patients had catheters in for more than 24 hours, she and her staff would have enough time to coordinate the care needed to ensure the catheters were removed and the risk of infection eliminated.

When Debbie and Laura looked at worker injury data and engaged with the staff on 4C, they learned that their injuries most often occurred when they were interrupted or distracted while performing an activity. To learn more about this so they could determine the right solutions, they decided to track the number of phone calls nurses received every hour. They thought that would be a great place to begin to understand more about interruptions and would be the first step toward eliminating high-risk activity resulting in worker injuries. Laura helped Debbie create a data collection plan in order to get more staff involved in the process and engaged in the discussions around eliminating patient and worker harm.

Sue, Cheryl, Laura, and Debbie continued to meet regularly until they had agreed upon measures for each of the True North goals of safety and quality, patient satisfaction, employee satisfaction, and sustainability. They knew they were setting up their areas to be successful by aligning the work they did every day to the True North of the organization and that their efforts to make their daily work better were directly contributing to making ABC Health System the best place to receive and provide care.

COLLABORATIVE CORNER
Holes in the Swiss Cheese

One way to think about the relationship between lagging and leading indicators is to imagine them as holes in slices of Swiss cheese. Each slice has multiple holes. When we stack up the slices, occasionally all of the holes line up and something slides through, which in clinical practice results in an adverse event or bad outcome (figure 5.2). Those adverse events are the lagging indicator that there was a problem. The holes that exist in every slice of Swiss cheese are the leading indicators that a vulnerability exists that could result in an adverse event. There are many more holes in the Swiss cheese than there are slices of cheese. If one can understand what and where the holes are in each slice of cheese, it means there are many more opportunities to prevent problems rather than waiting for the adverse event to happen. The impact on the outcome measures or lagging indicators can occur much faster if the process measures or leading indicators are focused on, understood, and improved every day.

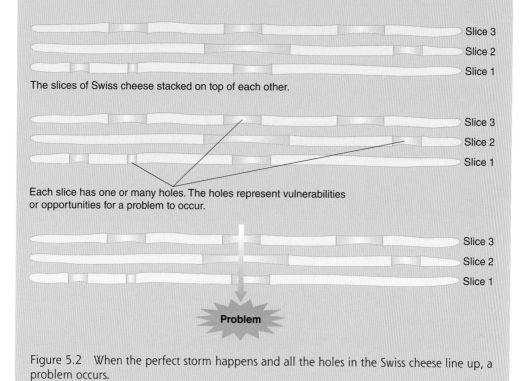

Figure 5.2   When the perfect storm happens and all the holes in the Swiss cheese line up, a problem occurs.

used as leading indicators. A key to effective leading indicators is keeping them easy to collect. Pen and paper and a quick tally or count taken as close to real time as possible is a great way to think of process measures. To ensure the information will be collected and stay current, the collection process should not add a lot of work for anyone engaged in gathering the data.

An example of a lagging indicator is falls. When measuring the number of falls that have occurred, the data reflect a count of events that have already happened; subsequently, the day-to-day improvement work at local levels in the organization will likely not show immediate improvement in the overall data. To determine an appropriate process measure, or leading indicator for falls, seek to understand what processes or workflows may contain a vulnerability that could lead to a fall. For instance, what is the standard for how often to ambulate patients? How does one know if that work is being done as designed? Is there a risk assessment that is standardized and understood for all to use, and is it being followed as intended (at the right point in the care process) in order to develop the right care plan for that patient? After engaging with the people who provide direct care to patients, decisions on process measures can be made. For example, an hour-by-hour count of bed alarms activated could be a valuable manual measure to provide information on the number of falls.

Constructing the Team

Given the history of certain health care professions, it can be easy to call the usual group members together and falsely assume that they represent the entirety of who is needed in order to comprehensively work on the problem. Historically, physicians and nurses have worked closely together, and in forming a health care team at an outpatient clinic one may inadvertently forget to include the office manager or a billing specialist for a goal that is directly or indirectly influenced by these team members. Likewise, in an acute care medical center, a health care group of physicians and nurses may neglect to include nursing assistants, RTs, case managers, and therapy services because the latter members are not a part of the traditional decision-making group. It is imperative that the team include representatives from all professions and disciplines engaged in the work (see figure 5.3).

To have all the appropriate health care providers engaged as team members, it is necessary to ensure that the people who do the work are the people who define the work processes. A nursing supervisor who does not provide bedside care may have a voice in the overall development of work processes but should defer to the nursing assistants or nurses regarding the details of the current workflow and work challenges at the bedside. Not only should all frontline health care providers be represented on the team, but it is essential for their perspectives to be equally valued, if not more highly valued, than those of the supervisors who are not directly engaged in the direct workflow. This engagement of the frontline direct care providers facilitates ecologically valid and valuable problem solving.

In business, the term **cross-boundary teaming** refers to individuals with differences in expertise and organization forming a temporary group tasked with quickly developing into an effective and efficient team to address a novel project.[12] This increased **knowledge diversity** on the team facilitates innovative thinking. However, according to Edmondson and Harvey, studies indicate that teaming across boundaries is particularly challenging, and they attribute this to people taking the norms and values of their own professions and organizations for granted.[12] Given the defined roles of health care professions, as well as the cultures within health care professions, teams can experience both the challenges and benefits of knowledge diversity.

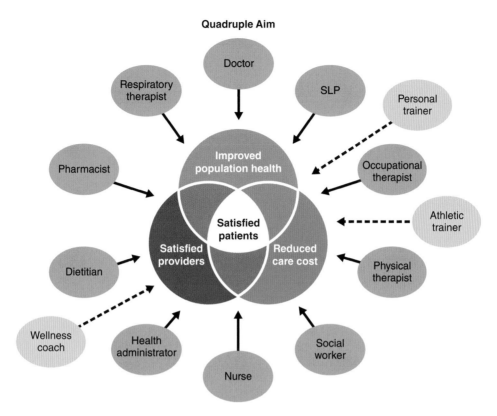

Figure 5.3 Quadruple Aim and interprofessional representation.

Gathering the Team

It is valuable to consider the logistical aspects of gathering a new or renovated team to ensure the ongoing participation of the people who are needed to work on the problem. For example, the meeting date, time, and frequency should allow all team members to attend without placing undue burden or stress on any one team member or type of professional. The burden of work during the day or shift can vary substantially among roles, so it is valuable to instill a sense of respect for all team members' schedules. Letting the team determine the schedule is a great way to demonstrate respect and ensure alignment around the time commitment needed; otherwise, this can be a barrier to open communication among the team members. One way to determine the schedule is to create an informal online survey to collect preferred days and times for the team. When considering scheduling logistics, try to make it easy, efficient, and worthwhile for all team members to attend. In practice areas that employ health care providers who provide 24-hour services, it may be valuable to hold **sister meetings** between day shifts and night shifts. Also, consider using technology to promote remote participation. The organizer should intentionally make the meeting accessible to all team members.

Interprofessional Professionalism

Although uncommon, a new health care team may be composed of people who are all new to one another and are starting their collaboration as equally new members of the team. In this instance, it is helpful to cooperatively establish norms for communication and decision making. Each team member brings personal and professional values, biases, and assumptions, which can affect the tone, pattern, and format of the teamwork.

Teams are formed to address a shared goal or set of goals, and effective teams are aligned by shared values in how to accomplish the goal. According to the Interprofessional Professionalism Collaborative (IPC),[13] **interprofessional professionalism** is the "consistent demonstration of core values evidenced by professionals working together, aspiring to and wisely applying principles of altruism, excellence, caring, ethics, respect, communication, accountability to achieve optimal health and wellness in individuals and communities."[14(p103)] The IPC developed a tool to assess a person's level of interprofessional professionalism, the Interprofessional Professionalism Assessment (IPA). This tool was developed for use with health care professionals who are in training, but it also could be used for team member assessment or for self-assessment to introduce and emphasize the core values of interprofessional professionalism for health professionals.[14]

Incorporating the IPCP core values into the patterns of workflow and communication in an established health care group can be a challenge. Given the history of health care and the multitude of health care roles, there is a commonly regarded hierarchy among providers. This historical hierarchy in health care can present a barrier to respectful collaboration among the interprofessional team members. In early team discussions and problem-solving efforts, it is recommended that the person responsible for assembling the team lead by example and set the standard for what respectful behaviors are expected in the group. There may be a need for members of the team who traditionally give orders to practice humble inquiry in order to seek additional information or understanding. Additionally, those who receive orders may need to be drawn out in the conversations and be empowered to share ideas. Effective facilitation is critical to achieving an effective group dynamic. All members are responsible for showing respect to others and for creating a culture of psychological safety.

In a work environment, such as in health care, **psychological safety** refers to the perceived consequences of taking interpersonal risks.[3] Edmondson and Lei explain that psychological safety promotes employees' willingness to engage in a shared effort though taking the initiative to contribute their ideas.[16] A sequence of studies concluded that psychological safety is a group-level phenomenon, and groups within the same organization can vary notably with regard to this perception of consequences. In a team, there are many factors that can influence the level of psychological safety:

- The power within the broader organization, either formal or informal, that any member of the team has
- The historical relationship between or perception of various departments and services within an organization
- Individual relationships that exist

TOOLS OF IPE
Practicing Humble Inquiry to Develop Capability and Empower Team Members

As leaders, facilitators, and teammates, it is imperative to understand how the types of questions we ask can influence the interactions we have. Following are 4 types of questions from Edgar Schein:

1. *Humble inquiry*—The purpose is to seek to understand with no ulterior motives or judgment, asking almost childlike questions. This respects the work that has already been done and shows sincere interest in the thoughts of the person being asked. The major role of the person asking this type of question is to actively listen to the response in order to better know what questions to ask.

2. *Diagnostic inquiry*—The purpose is for the question to help the answerer see or learn the cause-and-effect relationships in the information they are thinking about and to dig deeper in understanding the problem. It is not about what the asker of questions knows; it is about the person being asked the questions learning how to find the answer.

3. *Prompting inquiry*—This is sometimes called *confrontational inquiry*. It is often done with the best of intentions but builds or maintains dependency on the person asking the questions because the questioner is inserting ideas and not challenging the answerer with thinking through and coming up with ideas. The questions are prompted by the asker's own thinking and therefore infuse the same bias into the process.

4. *Coaching process inquiry*—The purpose is to force reflection on a shared interaction with the intent to build the relationship between the asker and answerer. The question asker can learn what about the process or experience was most helpful and what to improve for future interactions.[15]

It is important to understand the 4 kinds of questions, but in order to develop capability and empower team members, the focus should be on humble inquiry. Here are some tips for practicing humble inquiry in a group setting:

- Ask questions and listen with sincere interest to the answers.
- Practice the power of the pause: Ask a question and then wait. Allow 10 seconds after asking a question before speaking again so people have the space to answer. People need time to think in order to formulate thoughtful responses.
- Make sure all members are given an opportunity to share their insights. All voices are needed in order to fully understand situations and minimize bias; no two perspectives are completely the same.
- Reinforce that the experts are the people who do the work and that their voices are critical to understanding the total picture and what to do.

It is important to understand the factors that can influence the psychological safety of a team because it directly correlates with group performance. Furthermore, cooperation and a climate of trust promote a problem-solving orientation for the group, including team members sharing and learning from one another's mistakes.[16] Therefore, it is valuable to invest in creating a team culture with psychological safety to promote team collaboration, problem solving, and success.

Creating Psychological Safety

When promoting psychological safety within a group, it can be helpful to consider differing perspectives and levels of team members' psychological and emotional comfort. Consider the following questions to reflect on key aspects of team culture:

- Do all team members feel safe in relation to gender, race, and ethnicity?
- Is team communication accessible to all members (e.g., members with visual or hearing impairments)?
- Is there respect for team members' emotional well-being? For example, has team leadership mitigated the risk of a member being aggressive or manipulative?

When establishing psychological safety, it is necessary to establish healthy patterns of communication and behavior through reinforcement in communications and through modeling behavior that aligns with the following values.

- Focus on the facts of what has happened or is happening. Speak from the voice of the process and not the people involved in the process.
- Clarify roles for select team members, and allow team roles to be dynamic. The same person does not always have to serve the same role for the team. Positions have definitive start and end dates to promote leadership development and opportunity for all interested team members. Some examples of roles are the following:
  - Agenda setter (sent beforehand to keep focus during the meeting)
  - Minute taker (sent afterward so everyone can keep up with what was discussed, accomplished, and needed for next time)
  - Logistics coordinator (administrative support to help schedule the meeting)
  - Facilitator (meeting leader who keeps the meeting on task, on time, and focused)
  - Presenter or liaison to leadership (for updates)
  - Live note taker (using flip chart and markers during meetings)
- Verbalize the value of beginning and ending team meetings on time, and commit to effective meeting management by adhering to the times that have been agreed upon by the group. Even if it means stopping a conversation before it is complete, it is important to adhere to the agreed-upon times. Respect for time is a great way to show respect for people. This allows team members to be less stressed about being late to another work obligation.
- Clearly state the importance of nonpunitive problem solving and discussions. If a team member shares about learning from an error, then the focus of the

dialogue is on sharing the learning and the processes involved. Without exception, people should never be the root cause of any problem.

- Kindly reinforce the value of remaining focused on productive dialogue rather than superfluous conversations. As needed, regularly return the dialogue to the central problem or concern. If new information is being brought to the fore that may not align with the current work or topic, using a shared list of notes, called a *parking lot*, can be an effective way to honor the information being shared while keeping the group on task. Parking lots should always be cleared at the end of a meeting to understand who will continue investigating those topics or give a timeline for further discussion if the topics are unable to be pursued at the current time.
- Encourage team members to practice noticing when their biases may be impeding their openness to new ideas.
- Remind team members that thinking outside the box is more likely to lead to new solutions, so innovative ideas are accepted and valued as a part of the team's problem solving.

The team members may also elect to use established patterns for communication, which could be as formal as **Robert's Rules of Order** or as simple as raising a hand to indicate the wish to share an insight. The priority is that the pattern of communication is healthy and supports the established team values.

Characteristics of an Effective Team Member

A survey of more than 200 members in the Australian College of Health Service Executives indicated that the most highly ranked attributes of members of health care management teams were the following: commitment to collaborative work, commitment to a quality outcome, and commitment to organization.[17]

Characteristics of effective team members are diverse because an effective team thrives when there are different personalities and perspectives. There is value in having team members who are naturally curious as well as those who prefer to wait and see. Diversity in a group will promote a well-rounded perspective shared among the team regarding the organization as a whole. For teams that represent organizations or initiatives within an organization, it is valuable to seek out formal and informal leaders as well as attract team members who are willing to try new ideas, also called *early adopters*.

When using change management tools to plan for the best way to implement changes, there are 3 types of people to consider:

1. *Actively welcome change*—People who actively welcome change are early adopters, and they will always raise their hand first to try new things and contribute to new ideas. Early adopters are the team members who are eager to test new ideas, processes, or tools.

2. *Passively comply with change*—Those who passively comply with change like to wait and see. They watch with interest how the changes are happening and reserve support until they see the results. People who wait and see need the concepts and benefits proven to them before they support a change.

3. *Actively resist change*—Those who actively resist change, or laggards, openly speak out against change and lag behind the group in adopting new practices regardless of the change or how it is communicated.

Team Development and Redevelopment

When developing a health care team, it is important to reflect on Bruce Tuckman's model of group development. Tuckman proposes that small groups undergo the following 5 stages:

1. Forming (testing and dependence)
2. Storming (intragroup conflict)
3. Norming (development of group cohesion)
4. Performing (functional role relatedness)
5. Adjourning[18]

When applying this model to health care teams, consider that it is more common to have ongoing team activities over many phases of problems that require collaborative problem solving over an extended time, and in some cases members are functioning 24 hours a day. It is understandable that health care teams do not always follow Tuckman's model neatly. Therefore, new membership may require the group to return to an earlier phase in the model; it may feel more like the team is forming or storming again after experiencing the performing stage. Other authors note that new team members will look to the veteran team members for guidance on roles and norms and will try to develop a sense of belonging.[12] These authors further highlight that newcomers will try to influence the team dynamics for developing their fit within the team. Greeting newcomers and losing members is an inherent challenge and benefit of long-term health care teams. Team members can emphasize the benefit by welcoming the newcomer's knowledge and providing the newcomer with information on team norms for ease of assimilation.

Work groups that are formed to solve a specific problem in the organization are often charged with achieving a specific outcome and are expected to immediately make an impact. They are quickly formed and instantly begin to focus on their charge as a group. The group often has aggressive deadlines because it was formed in response to outcomes that are being tracked, which reveal the need for improvements and require a concerted effort to address. Frequently when work groups are formed, there is little or no emphasis placed on how they develop as a team. They are chosen, brought together, and unleashed. The problem is that all teams go through stages (forming, storming, norming, and performing) when they come together to tackle a specific task, and these stages influence the ability to focus on or deliver the necessary results. All teams go through this process in some part, and the speed with which the team advances through the stages affects how long it takes to get to the optimal stage, performing.

Taking the time to bring a group of people together in order to acknowledge and help them through the challenges of each stage of development accelerates the team's ability to provide results. When results are needed immediately, there is no

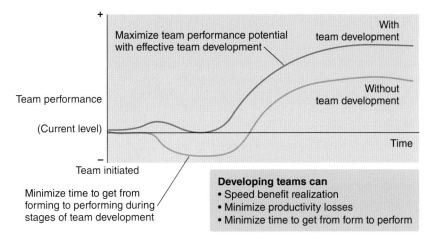

Figure 5.4 Team development and productivity.

time to waste. Time, or lack thereof, plays a big role in the development of a work group. What many people fail to see is the impact of time spent on development on the overall time it takes to go from forming to performing. Any amount of time a team attempts to cut from the initial development stages will be spent tenfold later in the process, affecting not only how quickly the team transitions to performing but also the level of performing the team can ultimately achieve (figure 5.4).

Collaboration Tools and Team Activities

Several team-building tools and QI methodologies exist to facilitate IPCP and team activities. As previously mentioned, teams are initiated to address a shared goal or set of goals. Within health care, these goals often focus on patient quality outcomes or safe clinical practice needs that warrant problem solving and are heavily dependent on intrapersonal and interpersonal awareness.

Interprofessional Professionalism Assessment

As discussed earlier, the IPA is a standardized tool that was developed by the IPC, a body composed of 12 entry-level health professions and a medical education assessment organization.[14] This tool was developed for use with health care professionals in training, such as students completing clinical education rotations or entry-level providers in their orientation.[14] The assessment is available on the IPC website at no cost. It measures 6 areas of professionalism: altruism and caring, excellence, ethics, respect, communication, and accountability. The individual items on the assessment provide succinct descriptions of behaviors of interprofessional professionalism. The IPA is an excellent foundation for providing feedback to the entry-level health care provider or student and for reflecting on and demonstrating these behaviors for developing interprofessional professionalism.

Team Oriented Problem Solving

Team Oriented Problem Solving (TOPS) is a multifaceted problem-solving strategy that requires at minimum 4 participants from 4 organizational areas who methodically apply 8 disciplines (8D) to solve a problem:

1. Form the team.
2. Define the problem.
3. Implement interim containment actions (ICAs).
4. Define problem root causes.
5. Develop permanent corrective actions.
6. Implement permanent corrective actions.
7. Prevent reoccurrences.
8. Recognize and congratulate the team.[19]

The TOPS methodology uses problem-solving tools from QI and project management fields, such as process mapping, prioritization matrices, and fishbone diagrams.[20] Following the conclusion of the 8 disciplines, TOPS facilitator teams recommend internal publication of problem-solving findings and pertinent highlights or lessons learned. Organizations typically focus on steps 1 through 3 when solving problems. This is called *firefighting* and is the extent of the problem-solving capability that exists in some organizations. It can be thought of as have need, meet need. For some team members, their entire roles may be designed around meeting the needs, or fighting the fires, that arise each day.

The difference between an organization focusing on steps 1 through 3 and one that fully uses the TOPS methodology can be understood in a simple example. Imagine a supply frequently used in clinical practice that a clinician has to look for in various places before finding it, such as alcohol wipes. If Ida the nurse is administering a flu shot, she needs an alcohol wipe to prep the vaccination site before injection. If Ida attempts to give a patient an injection but finds her workstation container is empty of wipes, she leaves her immediate workstation and goes to the next room. If she finds wipes there, she brings a handful back to her own workstation and administers the vaccination. Ida is able to meet the current need (administer the vaccination), but does she solve the root cause of the problem? Will she have this problem again? Will someone else? How many times do clinicians find what they need the first place they look for it? How many times do they have to look in multiple places before finding what they need? How many times do they not find what they need and have to call to another department to get it? The difference between typical problem solving and TOPS is the difference between solving the problem of "need alcohol wipe, get alcohol wipe" daily and "need alcohol wipe, do something so that everyone who needs an alcohol wipe always has one when they need it, where they need it" so that they never have to solve that problem again.

Scientific Method to Solve Problems

The scientific method is ingrained in clinicians; it is learned and practiced and part of every activity every day. A crucial way to accelerate the ability of an organization to solve problems quickly is to develop the ability to apply the scientific method to all problems, all the time. In clinical work, one always practices the scientific method. For instance, conducting a history and physical assessment with a patient follows the scientific method, and any clinician can explain the steps. When clinicians are asked how to solve a process problem they experience, however, they inevitably circumvent the scientific method and jump to a solution without proper observation, assessment, and measurement. Clinical leaders need to train their brains to apply the scientific method to solving problems other than patients' conditions. Using the scientific method ensures that a repeatable (and therefore, teachable) process is being used to think through problems and solve them at the root cause.

Lean Methodology

Another robust problem-solving method that supports interprofessional team development and collaboration is Lean. Lean methodology focuses on quality health care, patient safety, and service improvement by reducing errors by removing waste (steps or tasks that don't add value), facilitating IPCP, and eliminating barriers to safe patient care.[21]

A3 is a problem-solving tool in Lean methodology whereby team members evaluate their workflows and environments with a new perspective focused on system-level vulnerabilities rather than personal vulnerabilities.[21] An A3 leads participants through a structured evaluation of problem, need, background, associated measures, and current state using a 5-whys questioning process before ever thinking about a solution. The 5 whys reveal system-level vulnerabilities and eliminate blame on personal practices or skills (figure 5.5).

Problem: Need: Background:	Ideal:			
Measures:	Hypotheses:			
Current state and 5 whys:	Action items:			
	What?	Who?	When?	Y/N
	Key learnings:			

Figure 5.5   Lean methodology: A blank A3 tool.

Aligned with psychological safety, a core element of Lean methodology that differs from traditional top-down change management is the recognition that problem solving and QI are informed and defined by the people who do the work.[21] Within health care, this commitment strengthens IPCP by ensuring all relevant clinicians are represented during patient safety and QI discussions. In addition, in Lean methodology problems are addressed with rapid experimentation, experimentation is collaborative, and team members at all levels of an organization are involved in experiments.

Six Sigma

Another QI strategy that may be used to support IPCP is Six Sigma, a philosophy and methodology used to reduce or remove identifiable sources of variation that result in defective outputs in order to ensure only small levels of random variation remain. Given that this strategy focuses on developing highly standardized processes and that variation is inherent in providing patient-centered care, Six Sigma is recommended for standard work processes that do not warrant adaptations or variations among patients.[22]

EBP OF TEAMSHIP
Evidence Based Strategies for Improving Teamwork

In a study protocol article, O'Leary and colleagues define their current research on redesigning clinical microsystems in order to improve teamwork and quality of patient care in the hospital environment. This research team defines the clinical microsystem as a "small group of people who work together in a defined setting on a regular basis to provide care."[24(p2)]

This research effort systematically applies evidence-based individual strategies for improving teamwork, and therefore quality of patient care, in a standardized, comprehensive, and unified manner at 4 hospitals in the United States. The researchers call the unified list of inventions used in their study the *Advanced and Integrated MicroSystems (AIMS)* interventions, which include unit-based physician teams, unit nurse–physician coleadership, enhanced interprofessional rounds, unit-level performance reports, and patient engagement activities.

The primary outcome measures for this research will be rate of adverse events and teamwork climate, as assessed by the Safety Attitudes Questionnaire (SAQ). The secondary outcome measures will be efficiency, defined by median length of stay and by 30-day readmissions, and the patient experience using the Hospital Consumer Assessment of Healthcare Providers and Systems (HCAHPS) global ratings of hospital care.[24]

Summary

IPCP involves "multiple health workers from different professional backgrounds working together with patients, families, caregivers, and communities to deliver the highest quality of care."[8(p7)] When planning an interprofessional team, identifying a meaningful common goal for the group is the foundation for assembling members. The goal should be tied directly to the strategic plan of the organization and the True North goals that the organization is working to achieve. It is imperative that the team include representation from all professions and disciplines engaged in the work. The people who do the work should be the people who define the work (patient care) processes to facilitate ecologically valid and valuable problem solving. This collaboration ensures knowledge diversity on the team and facilitates innovative thinking.[12]

Several team-building tools and QI methodologies exist to facilitate IPCP and team activities:

- IPA is a standardized tool used to measure 6 areas of professionalism (altruism and caring, excellence, ethics, respect, communication, and accountability) to prepare clinicians to exhibit these behaviors for interprofessional professionalism development.

- TOPS is a multifaceted problem-solving strategy that requires at minimum 4 participants from 4 organizational areas who methodically apply 8 disciplines (8D).

- Lean methodology centers on quality health care, patient safety, and service improvement by reducing errors by removing waste, facilitating IPCP, and eliminating barriers to safe patient care.

- Six Sigma is a QI philosophy and methodology used to reduce or remove identifiable sources of variation that result in defective outputs in order to ensure only small levels of random variation remain.

This chapter has emphasized the importance of the team construct. Chapter 6 will present a more detailed overview of the development of effective teams, their leadership, and application to support IPCP.

CASE STUDY Debriefing

Kevin, Christine, and Marie want to start a new project on bathroom safety with the Fall Champions. Organizational data indicate that 25% of patient falls with injury occur in the bathroom, and several falls have resulted in significant injury. They need to bring a team together to ensure the people doing the work are the people defining the work, and they need to present an action plan to executive leaders in the next 6 weeks.

Case Study Discussion Questions

1. What team members should Kevin, Christine, and Marie include in the interprofessional group focused on bathroom safety?
2. What team-building activities could they include to foster team development (forming, storming)?
3. What QI method should they use to focus on root causes of falls in the bathroom?
4. What leading and lagging measures could they consider measuring?

CHAPTER 6

Teaming to Achieve Patient and Organizational Outcomes

Robin Dennison, DNP, APRN, CCNS, NEA-BC
Amy Herrington, DNP, RN, CEN, CNE
Melanie Logue, PhD, DNP, APRN, CFNP, FAANP

Objectives

After reading this chapter, the reader will be able to do the following:

- Describe the significance of interprofessional teamwork, teams, and teaming to patient and organizational outcomes.
- Discuss the relationship between IPE and effective interprofessional teams.
- Apply best practices related to team structure.
- Relate effective interprofessional teaming to patient and organizational outcomes.
- Provide examples of strategies for interprofessional teamwork.

CASE STUDY A Simple Procedure

Mrs. Jones is a 63-year-old with a history of osteoarthritis. She has had difficulty ambulating for 10 years, but as the primary caregiver for her husband, she has been unable to have a total hip replacement. Since her husband's death 6 months ago, Mrs. Jones' mobility has drastically declined. She now ambulates with a walker. Additionally, she has been depressed and has not been eating well. Her children visit infrequently because they live 400 miles (644 km) away.

Following an evaluation by Dr. Patel, Mrs. Jones is scheduled for a total hip replacement. Dr. Patel has been caring for Mrs. Jones for 10 years and is keenly aware

(continued)

Case Study (continued)

of her orthopedic deterioration. Due to their long-standing relationship, he evaluates Mrs. Jones in the office and determines that no preadmission testing is needed for the procedure. Mrs. Jones is told to expect 2 days of hospitalization and then discharge to home with outpatient physical therapy. She is encouraged by the plan.

Mrs. Jones' surgery proceeds as scheduled. Unfortunately, she experiences quite a bit of intraoperative blood loss and requires transfusion. She is transferred to telemetry afterward for monitoring.

During the first postoperative hours, Mrs. Jones develops shortness of breath. Dr. Patel attributes this to atelectasis due to lack of ambulation, and he asks the nursing staff to get Mrs. Jones out of bed and take her for a walk in the hallway. However, this request is never implemented because Mrs. Jones resists efforts to assist her with ambulation.

Nurse Choi, Mrs. Jones' primary nurse, has profound concerns about caring for her. She is a cardiac nurse and has never taken care of a patient after a total hip replacement. Additionally, she is confused on bed mobility. Nurse Choi calls the PT, who refuses to see Mrs. Jones because Dr. Patel has not requested a consult. He tells Nurse Choi that he will evaluate Mrs. Jones when prescribed by the doctor.

Ms. Lunsford, the dietitian, completes routine screening on all postsurgical patients. She becomes concerned when she determines that Mrs. Jones reported a 20-lb (9-kg) weight loss on admission. However, she is now 5 lb (2 kg) heavier than she was preoperative. The dietitian notes that Mrs. Jones has difficulty speaking due to shortness of breath.

As the next day progresses, Mrs. Jones is not ready to go home. Due to conflicting roles and poor communication, she is never moved out of bed. Though her shortness of breath improves with a diuretic, she has never ambulated and has now developed a pressure ulcer on her coccyx. The family is called by the social worker to arrange for home care.

The social worker learns during the meeting with the family that no one can care for Mrs. Jones at home, so arrangements are made for long-term care. Mrs. Jones becomes depressed and withdrawn. She worries that she will never leave the nursing home. She worries that no one will take care of Clementine, her basset hound.

As health care professionals, our primary goals are to optimize patient and organizational outcomes. These goals are not achieved in isolation; they are best achieved through effective teaming. Teaming is an active process of working together.[1] This chapter will discuss the significance of **interprofessional teamwork**, **teams**, and **teaming**; the relationship between IPE and effective interprofessional teams; best practices for team structure; the effect of teaming on patient and organizational outcomes; and specific strategies for interprofessional teamwork.

Health Care Teaming

Cohen and Bailey define a *team* as "a collection of individuals who are interdependent in their tasks, who share responsibility for outcomes, who see themselves and who are seen by others as an intact social entity embedded in one or more larger social systems (for example, business unit or corporation), and who manage their relationships across organizational boundaries."[2(p241)] A team is simply a group of people working together to complete a job, task, or project with a mutual goal. If this team consists of health care providers, the focus is on multiple functions and goals, such as optimizing patient or organizational outcomes as well as creating a healthy workplace. A key function of health care teams for achieving these goals is interprofessional teamwork.

Teams are not a new concept, but they are more important than ever thanks to initiatives such as the Triple Aim.[3] Whether or not an interprofessional team is effective also needs to be determined. Effective interprofessional health care teams are characterized by "positive leadership and management attributes; communication strategies and structures; personal rewards, training and development; appropriate resources and procedures; appropriate skill mix; supportive team climate; individual characteristics that support interdisciplinary team work; clarity of vision; quality and outcomes of care; and respecting and understanding roles."[4(p1)] These characteristics have been revised into the following 10 competencies for an effective team:

1. Identifies a leader who establishes a clear direction and vision for the team while listening and providing support and supervision to the team members.

2. Incorporates a set of values that clearly provide direction for service provision by the team; these values should be visible and consistently portrayed.

3. Demonstrates a team culture and interdisciplinary atmosphere of trust where contributions are valued and consensus is fostered.

4. Ensures appropriate processes and infrastructures are in place to uphold the vision of the service (e.g., referral criteria, communications infrastructure).

5. Provides quality patient-focused services with documented outcomes; uses feedback to improve quality of care.

6. Uses communication strategies that promote intrateam communication, collaborative decision making, and effective team processes.

7. Provides sufficient team staffing to integrate an appropriate mix of skills, competencies, and personalities to meet the needs of patients and enhance functioning.

8. Facilitates recruitment of staff members who demonstrate interdisciplinary competencies, including team functioning, collaborative leadership, communication, and sufficient professional knowledge and experience.

9. Promotes role interdependence while respecting individual roles and autonomy.

10. Facilitates personal development through appropriate training, rewards, recognition, and opportunities for career development.

EBP OF TEAMSHIP
Who Can Lead *Your* Team?

As the 10 competencies suggest, it is important to identify and appoint the right leader. Leadership styles, personality traits, and experience are all things to consider when establishing this role. We have all worked with various types of leaders and perhaps have read about the differences between bosses versus leaders. A skilled leader can help a team to work effectively and efficiently while moving the group toward the end goal. Defining values and expectations upfront is useful in setting the tone for group work. Building psychological trust and inclusion is also valuable in creating a culture to uphold the vision and mission of the team. Diversity is recognized and communication is essential to promote satisfaction and attainment of goals. We have all worked in teams that have been highly productive and those that have not. Think about what characteristics made your team function well or hindered its functioning. List those characteristics and how they relate to the 10 competencies for effective interprofessional health care teams. What might you change or continue moving forward with?

Edmondson has coined the term *teaming* to refer to an active process of working together. She suggests that teaming blends the following:

- Relating to people
- Listening to other points of view
- Coordinating actions
- Sharing decision making[1]

Teaming blends both **affective skills** and **cognitive skills**. Interprofessional teams blend the affective and cognitive skills of multiple professions to optimize organizational and patient outcomes.

Why are interprofessional teams important? Many research studies have found improved patient and organizational outcomes with effective interprofessional teamwork (see chapter 4 for a summary of this work). The IPEC Expert Panel has written that "evidence suggests that interprofessional teams achieve better outcomes and that **interprofessional team-based care** should become the normative clinical practice."[5(p11)] The NAM Committee on the Health Professions Education recommends that "all health professionals should be educated to deliver patient-centered care as members of an interdisciplinary team, emphasizing evidence-based practice, quality improvement, and informatics."[6(p18)]

However, Vega and Bernard contend that interprofessional teamwork is the exception rather than the rule in health care. Each health care profession cannot operate in silos but must shift toward collaboration. Quality, safety, and cost effectiveness require mutual respect and collaboration. The authors also emphasize the importance of interprofessional teamwork for efficiency, which is necessary due to the projected shortage of health care providers and the increasing need for health care by the aging population.[7]

Interprofessional teams may collaborate in different ways using different models.

- Figure 6.1 illustrates a model of interprofessional teamwork to facilitate patient care. In this scenario, a patient is admitted to a department and is assigned a small interprofessional team who collaborates on the patient's care until discharge.

- Figure 6.2 illustrates a different approach. In this model, team-based care operates on a continuum, pulling in interprofessional team members as their expertise is needed or as the care plan requires. Notice the presence of family in both models of interprofessional team-based care; the dotted line indicates the involvement of family from intake to discharge.

- Figure 6.3 advances model 2 by highlighting how an interprofessional care team might communicate regarding patient care. Notice the dotted lines indicating collaboration and sharing of information across the team members to facilitate patient care. Based on the patient's diagnosis and care needs, associated health care providers would be represented in this interprofessional team-based care schema.

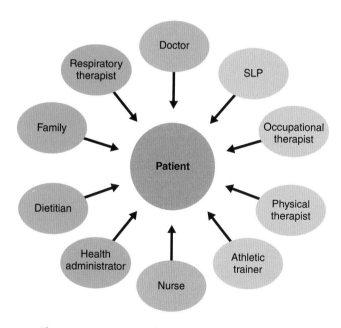

Figure 6.1   Interprofessional teamwork model 1.

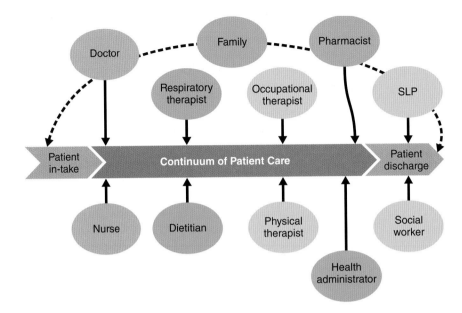

Figure 6.2   Interprofessional teamwork model 2.

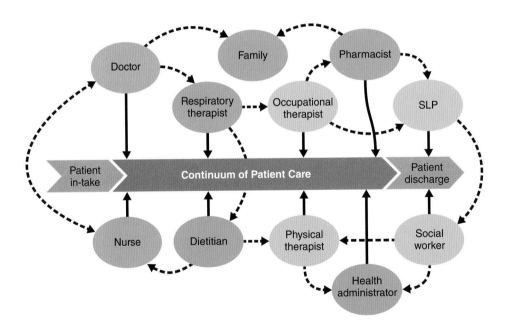

Figure 6.3   Interprofessional collaborative care communication.

TOOLS OF IPE
Inventory of Reflective Vignette
Interprofessional Learning (IRV-IPL)

This tool measures interprofessional learning by generating consistently reproducible results in areas such as collaboration, coordination, cooperation, communication, and commendation. It measures the ability of health care team members to work together, which may translate to team learning outcomes and eventually practice. Health care workers are expected to function cohesively under shared leadership, decision making, and accountability. The IRV-IPL measures interprofessional learning in continuing professional development, which makes it unique. It was developed after extensive literature review and designed with 3 segments to assess interprofessional competencies before, during, and after using vignettes.[31]

A key strategy for developing interprofessional teams and collaboration is IPE. WHO asserts that the primary intent of IPE is to prepare a collaborative-ready health workforce.[8] Improved communication and collaboration by interprofessional teams leads to better patient outcomes.[9] The Joint Commission has identified leadership, communication, coordination, and human factors as the root cause of errors in health care classified as sentinel events.[10] Increasingly, schools have sought to focus on these root causes with the integration of simulation or team training techniques and development programs. Competence to practice safely requires not only clinical expertise but also effective communication with patients and colleagues as well as family members and significant others.[11]

Teams

Teams have an explicit or implicit purpose, and they must include key stakeholders related to the purpose. The leadership and structure of the team are crucial to its success in meeting its purpose.

Purpose of a Team

Teams may be relatively permanent or temporary depending on their purpose. The focus of work teams is the mission of the organization, such as the provision of patient care. Although these teams are permanent, their membership changes over time. Various support teams provide assistance to others in fulfilling the mission of the organization. Ad hoc or project teams are temporary; they disband when their assigned work is complete.[12]

Development of a Team

The first step in creating a team is to provide a framework for it. This includes the purpose and goals of the team, expected deliverables, available resources, and accountability. There is also a need to create a safe environment for team members and their work.[13]

Selection of Team Members

The person or group creating the team needs to determine the KSAs (knowledge, skills, and attitudes), background, and expertise needed for success.[12] An ideal interprofessional team includes representatives of each profession that is a stakeholder in the team expectations; however, consideration must be given to size. Team size is related to function. A team that is too small will likely put too much pressure on each team member, whereas a team that is too large makes processes and decision making difficult. A common block to quality decision making in teams is groupthink.[14] Diverse membership is crucial, but so is provision of safety in the expression of each member's views. The team leader establishes the culture that offers safety for the expression of divergent views.

Structure of a Team

Structure and function are also aspects of defining a team. *Structure* refers to the composition of the team and is part of the teamwork process.[13] A properly structured care team enables effective communication, leadership, situation monitoring, and mutual support. Proper team structure can promote teamwork by including a clear leader, involving the patient, and ensuring that all team members commit to their roles in effective teamwork.

Many lessons can be taken from team sports. Teams are constructed with a goal in mind. Building a comprehensive program requires careful consideration of the team structure and function. Teams can be structured in numerous configurations to include variations in size, roles, types of professionals, and so on. Structure is the basic unit of team performance; it affects function, which affects process. The sum of the average team performance determines success or failure.[15] Some teams have certain structural requirements to pursue a goal while coordinating efforts. The team leader can influence performance and cohesion when interaction or interdependency is required as part of the team function.[15] The leader's influence, or coaching style, has been measured where team members have specific roles that are not always interchangeable. Team structure can also be hierarchal or nonhierarchal.

The military offers another perspective on team structure and performance. Rapidly developing technology has introduced unprecedented complexity into health care as we know it today. Teams have replaced individuals to accomplish complex tasks. Because poor team performance has dire consequences, the military has studied ways to improve team outcomes.[16] The term *team structure* often describes work in subtasks. The assignment of these subtasks requires the individual to be able to perform the task.

COLLABORATIVE CORNER
Team Development

Tuckman initially identified 4 stages of team development[18] and then later revised the process to 5 stages (see chapter 5):[19]

1. Forming
2. Storming
3. Norming
4. Performing
5. Adjourning

How would you as a team member consider these stages in the development of a team? Identify a behavior that would exemplify each stage (i.e., forming, storming, norming, performing, and adjourning).

The members of a health care team bring a range of expertise to the patient care experience. Members have differing perspectives, skills, and experience. Patients, family members, and other stakeholders ideally participate as members of a health care team.[17]

Team Collaboration

Morley and Cashell describe health care collaboration as "participation of patients, family, and a diverse team of often highly specialized healthcare professionals. Involvement of all these team members in a cooperative and coordinated way is essential to providing exceptional care."[17(p207)] Common themes in the literature suggest that "collaboration is an integration of activities and knowledge that requires a partnership of shared authority and responsibility."[17(p208)] Sullivan describes 4 elements that constitute collaborative practice in health care:

1. Coordination (i.e., working to achieve shared goals)
2. Cooperation (i.e., contributing to the team, understanding and valuing the contributions of other team members)
3. Shared decision making (i.e., relying on negotiation, communication, openness, trust, and a respectful power balance)
4. Partnerships (i.e., open, respectful relationships cultivated over time in which all members work equitably together)[20]

Research shows that collaborative teamwork leads to reduced length of hospital stay, improved compliance with standards, improved quality measures, and

TOOLS OF IPE
TeamSTEPPS Teamwork
Perceptions Questionnaire (T-TPQ)

This 50-item questionnaire measures attitudes and experiences in health care teams. It is a self-reported measure of teamwork within a department or organization. One measure in the tool captures how an individual approaches team-related issues. T-TPQ is based on the core components of teamwork that compose TeamSTEPPS: team structure, leadership, communication, mutual support, and situation monitoring. Scoring can be done in two ways: A total score may be calculated for each construct or summing of scores, which allows for more accurate statistical testing and is the preferred method for performing data analyses, or an average score may be computed for each construct. Change can occur in team function and may be reflected in a pretest–posttest design.[32]

improved symptom and psychosocial management[23] (see additional supportive findings in chapter 4). The consensus among health care experts is that collaborative practice will be more effective, efficient, and considerate of team roles.[17]

According to Morley and Cashell, instruments designed to measure collaboration often focus on interactions between specific professions, individual disciplines, or highly specific teams.[17] Other tools focus on assessing quality of IPE rather than team behaviors. The following tools have been published with some psychometric analysis:

- Index of Interdisciplinary Collaboration (IIC)
- Multidisciplinary Collaboration instrument (MDC)
- Interprofessional Perception Scale (IPS)
- Role Perception Questionnaire (RPQ), generic form
- University of the West of England Interprofessional Questionnaire (UWE-IP)
- Modified IIC
- Assessment of Interprofessional Team Collaboration Scale (AITCS)

Key Determinants of Collaboration

Key determinants of collaboration include the "opportunity, ability, and willingness of team members to work with the team in a collaborative way."[17(p212)]

Opportunity

The physical environment in which a team operates can affect collaborative interactions. Morley and Cashell suggest that "environment can be taken to include physical spaces, temporal arrangements, schedules, processes, organized activities, and communication tools that may either encourage or discourage effective team collaboration."[17(p212)] Work spaces and environments can either detract or promote team cohesion and collaboration. Distance, virtual, or asynchronous work spaces are examples of environments producing varied ability to collaborate.

Willingness

The psychological environment (i.e., attitudes and behaviors) at all levels is also a determinant of collaboration. Willingness to collaborate is affected by levels of group cohesion, constancy, education, previous experience, and personal maturity. Mutual trust and respect develop over time and are influenced by the perceived experience, education, and competence both of oneself and of other team members, which also influence the psychological environment. Finally, the ability to communicate efficiently and constructively influences respect and trust.[17]

Ability

Ability involves understanding role boundaries and expectations within the team. An approach that deemphasizes individual needs in favor of team goals may promote a more patient-centered model of care.[17] The ability to engage in effective negotiation and conflict resolution, use language of respect and dignity, and know what terminology to use with different professions is also key to effective and meaningful collaboration practices.

Barriers

Barriers to collaboration might include compensation, professional practice regulation, institutional policies, and the physical environment. Other internal factors might be in leadership and control of the team, as well as in varied interests, goals, expectations, styles, and experiences, all of which can impair communication and even generate conflict.[17]

Teaming and Outcomes

When exploring teaming, team building, and teamwork in health care, providers must begin with understanding the goals of the team. Teaming involves IPCP, which "occurs when multiple health workers and students from different professional backgrounds provide comprehensive health services by working with patients, their families, carers (caregivers) and communities to deliver the highest quality of care across settings."[8(p7)] In 2012, IOM met with stakeholders to begin work on reforming educational programs for health professionals operationalizing IPCP. The purpose of this work was to improve quality and safety for patients and drive a patient-centered model. It was quickly determined that no validated tool was being used to measure the relationship between IPE, IPCP, and patient outcomes.[21] A conceptual model was developed to address this deficit and is currently being used to evaluate programs and systems (see chapter 2).

The work of IOM (now known as NAM) is to transform collaborative practice in health care. Many economic, social, and technology changes are driving interprofessional teams to facilitate collaboration and communication. Specifically, health care leaders have begun to create models of care that include interprofessional teamwork. Other changes are driven by the ACA and include involving the patients as key members of the health care team, new payment systems, new models of care with a focus on primary care, population health and preventative medicine, and integrative health systems.[22]

Organizational Systems and Team Practice

Interprofessional team collaboration is expected to lead to substantial cost savings in the United States.[22] As we care for more people with chronic care conditions, these savings are directly tied to decreases in duplication of services, readmissions, ED visits, and patient morbidity. As in any industry, performance indicators are used to track and trend outcomes in order to drive change and improve costs and efficiency. This holds true in health care, specialty and accrediting agencies, and regulatory entities monitoring key performance indicators (KPIs). Overall performance directly relates to financial reimbursement and organizational survivability. KPIs are now seen as collaborative responsibilities that are not owned by any one profession. Outcomes are best reached through a team approach, with the various disciplines serving as checks and balances for team members.

As identified by WHO, the health care system faces the challenges of an aging workforce and complex care management.[8] IPCP is a team approach that should lead to improved health outcomes for individuals as well as international communities.

IPE and IPCP data analysis is a growing science. Early data published by Brandt and Lutfiyya demonstrate several trends when evaluating outcomes and the success of interprofessional systems and practice:

1. The redesign of the system is about changing the culture of care or education.
2. There is a need for strong leadership with a clear mission and vision.
3. Organizations must provide adequate resources for this transition process.
4. Systems must be developed to train individuals to practice collaboratively in place (practice), not just in didactic or simulated course offerings.
5. Establishing a direct cause-and-effect relationship between IPCP and patient outcomes is difficult.[22]

The evaluation of IPCP outcomes is a deliberate process and should involve an economist as well as other interdisciplinary team members to ascertain how the cost of education and resources offsets the patient and organizational outcomes that are achieved. Although outcomes assessment and management are a developing science, many organizations have published anecdotal and observational studies demonstrating outcomes.

Collaboration Between Two Health Systems

Health System A uses a complex medical home model for patients diagnosed with chronic health conditions as well as mental health disorders to manage the care of these high-cost, high-need patients. The model uses an interprofessional health care team and engages community and social services to manage the care of this at-risk patient population.

A competing organization, Health System B, developed a similar medical model and as a result noticed increasing numbers of patients using both systems. This led to the need to collaborate across health care systems and for the direct competitors to establish care coordination.[23]

The organizations worked together to create a concept map that began with identifying the patients who were using both systems. A root-cause analysis was conducted to determine why patients were seeking care outside one system and steps that would facilitate the partnership, shared infrastructure, team building, and comprehensive patient management.[23] Overall, there was a 28% decrease in ED visits, 50% decrease in inpatient admissions with the length of stay decreased by 49%, and 67% decrease in computed tomography (CT) scans. The gross charges decreased by 51%, with a 54% decrease in direct expenses. These changes represented a 71% increase in the operating margin.[23]

Community Partner Collaboration

Heart failure is a chronic, complex disease. Management of patients with heart failure requires collaboration with interprofessional partners to improve patient quality of life, decrease hospital readmissions, and decrease the overall cost of care. A rural hospital in the southeastern United States experienced profound Medicare penalties over a period of 3 years due to a high heart-failure readmission rate. As a result, an interprofessional team involving nurse leaders, pharmacists, providers, clinical nurses, and case managers developed a program following the Plan, Do, Study, Act process. Pharmacists collaborated with inpatient nursing staff on the management of patient medications and patient weight as well as provided discharge medication teaching. The pharmacists also collaborated with providers to ensure that medication discrepancies and nonadherence to clinical practice guidelines were addressed during inpatient care and treatment and again prior to patient discharge.[24]

Though only a modest decrease in hospital readmissions was experienced, patient satisfaction scores via HCAHPS (Hospital Consumer Assessment of Healthcare Providers and Systems) significantly increased. The organization also recognized that a population of patients with a secondary diagnosis of heart failure was not included in the project implementation and was included in hospital readmission data. Additionally, there was a need for organizational leadership support because staff members were pulled from the project due to reorganization.[24]

Cochrane Review of Outcomes

The evaluation of the impact of IPCP is a new science in which the search for the perfect tool to evaluate outcomes remains a difficult task. In a Cochrane review of 15 articles published between 1999 and 2011 focusing on IPE interventions involving multiple providers and the examination of patient outcomes, it was found that the most significant change was provider communication. Some studies focused on the improvement in mortality and morbidity, while others noted improvement in patient experience and satisfaction. Modest improvement after the creation of an interprofessional team was noted.[25]

In further review of these studies, education of team members was found to be the key focus.[25] Evaluation of sustained practice noted inconsistency; in health care, the reality is that the interprofessional team is not a consistent, stable unit. Team members leave and new members are added. Maintaining a consistent team with members who train together and then work together is difficult in the acute hospital setting. This supports previous theories that interprofessional training and education must be a component of the change in culture. Evaluation of outcomes must begin with evaluating the actions of the team to ensure consistent performance before evaluating the impact on patient outcomes.[26]

Strategies to Facilitate Teaming

Health care providers can use many strategies to facilitate communication and interprofessional teamwork. The goal of each strategy is to recognize the contribution each team member makes to the patient experience and the impact on patient outcomes. Additionally, IPCP enhances team and patient goal setting, drives quality, and facilitates holistic care.

Bedside Rounding

Bedside rounding is a deliberate process in which health care providers meet at the patient bedside to discuss goals, outcomes, daily care plans, and discharge plans. All team members involved in the care discuss what treatment will be delivered, how care will be delivered, and how team members will work with each other to achieve the goals. Most importantly, the dialogue allows the team members to gain an understanding of how care provided by other professionals influences care provided throughout the shift or stay. This allows for scheduling treatment and interventions to enhance the patient experience and allow for periods of rest and healing. A key member of the group is the patient, and patient input should drive the conversation and planning.

Operationalizing bedside rounding can be difficult if impromptu rounding occurs. As with other IPCP efforts, health care leaders must design systems in which rounding is a component of organizational culture. Providers should create a schedule with specific, predictable times for rounding. This allows all health care professionals to attend and family members to take part in the discussion.

Planning for Long-Term Care

The idea of interprofessional teamwork is not new to health care. For many years, long-term care facilities have engaged in planning sessions involving therapists, dietitians, nurses, case managers, unlicensed personnel, the patient, and family members. The meetings occur within 14 days of admission and then usually every 90 days thereafter. The purpose of these meetings is to set goals for rehabilitation and overall care. Additionally, patient preferences are explored and enveloped into the care plan, the discharge plan is developed, progress toward goals is assessed, and acute changes or declines are investigated. During the meeting, residents are encouraged to express concerns about their experience within the organization and share safety concerns. During annual accreditation visits, agents for Medicare review the minutes from these meetings to ascertain whether there is active problem solving and timely resolution of problems or concerns.

Huddles in Health Care

Many organizations have implemented interprofessional huddles. A huddle is "a short, stand-up meeting—10 minutes or less—that is typically used once at the start of each workday in a clinical setting. In inpatient units, the huddle takes place at the start of each major shift."[27(p18)] The purpose of the huddle is to allow staff members to actively manage quality and safety issues. The huddle is a time when interprofessional team members come together to discuss goals, barriers, and process-improvement initiatives. The huddles help staff members learn, plan, and work together to achieve the best patient outcomes.

To be successful, health care providers must learn to listen to all members of the team because each member possesses important patient information. Huddle leaders have the responsibility to engage all team members in the process of sharing information, observations, or concerns. It is through talking and listening to one another that problem solving occurs and change happens.[28]

Medical Home Models

In an effort to curb rising health care costs, the medical home model has gained new popularity. Initially created in 1967 as a tool to manage pediatric care,[30] the patient-centered medical home (PCMH) model is a team-based approach to providing health care using IPCP to address the holistic needs of the patient.[28] Combined with new technology tools, the interprofessional interaction can occur face to face or virtually, which brings patients and providers an unlimited flow of information and a venue for exchanging ideas and solving problems. The virtual exchange is especially important in regions that may be underserved, offering access to services

COLLABORATIVE CORNER
Using SIBR to Improve Patient Care

One model of rounding was developed by Dr. Joseph Stein of Emory University. Referred to as SIBR (structured interdisciplinary bedside rounds), the process was first modeled on stroke and internal medicine units.[29] The process involves spending 4 to 6 minutes on a physician introduction of the patient and sharing of daily care planning goals from each team member. Areas of concentration and concerns are addressed by team members, including pain management, overnight events, intake, output, nursing concerns, mobility, and discharge plans.[29] This program has been successful and is being modeled across the United States, Australia, and New Zealand. Reflecting on this model, it is easy to see how having physical therapists, OTs, staff nurses, discharge planners, case managers, dietitians, pharmacists, social workers, and neurologists simultaneously at the bedside of a patient who has suffered a stroke would improve communication, adherence to quality metrics and standards, and attainment of home and rehabilitation goals.

that may otherwise be limited, such as behavior health and nutrition services. Successful implementation can lead to the development of a plan to promote health and chronic disease management.[30]

This dynamic team approach has also proven to decrease the cost of care through the management of chronic conditions such as diabetes, as well as decreasing readmissions and ED visits. Cline, Sweeny, and Cooper report that after the establishment of a free clinic created following the PCMH structure, the number of ED visits did not decrease, but the number of admissions decreased by 70% and hospital readmissions decreased by 66%.[30] The cost savings attributed to the new model of care was $372,865, or about $4,000 per patient. Interestingly, the cost of running the free clinic was not considered when evaluating the cost savings the institution experienced.[30]

Summary

Effective interprofessional teamwork has been shown to improve patient and organizational outcomes. Health care education should incorporate IPE to produce a health care workforce that is ready for interprofessional teamwork. Organizations need to facilitate the development of team leaders and eliminate barriers to effective teaming. This chapter has discussed the significance of interprofessional teamwork, teams, and teaming; the relationship between IPE and effective interprofessional teams; best practices for team structure; the effect of teaming on patient and organizational outcomes; and specific strategies for interprofessional teamwork. The importance of communication in this process cannot be underscored, so chapter 7 will explore mechanisms of communication important to IPCP team functioning in clinical practice.

CASE STUDY Debriefing

It is clear that a breakdown in communication occurred in Mrs. Jones' case. Additionally, no staff member took ownership for Mrs. Jones. The staff members focused on "my job" instead of "our patient," which led to a failure to ambulate Mrs. Jones. As a result, Mrs. Jones suffered a pressure ulcer, prolonged hospitalization, and an overall poor outcome.

Case Study Discussion Questions

1. What cultural changes need to occur?
2. Should they be unit-based or organizational-based changes?
3. How would individual reprimands versus cultural change influence KPIs?
4. In creating an IPCP team, which health care professions would you include?
5. When would you involve the organization leader in the process?
6. What baseline data should be collected to ascertain the focus of the change?
7. What type of training would you implement for team members? Would this be just-in-time training? Formal classroom training? Workplace training?
8. What outcomes would you measure initially and moving forward?

CHAPTER 7

Interprofessional Communication Strategies

Dee M. Lance, PhD, CCC-SLP/L
Kim C. McCullough, PhD, CCC-SLP/L

Objectives

After reading this chapter, the reader will be able to do the following:

- Understand the components of communication in interprofessional teams.
- Use tools to identify effective communication techniques for interacting on interprofessional teams.
- Use communication to create a climate conducive to team building.
- Apply effective communication strategies to improve client care.

CASE STUDY Communication: What Went Wrong?

Bellerive Rehabilitation Center prides itself on its collaborative model of patient care. When a new patient is admitted, there is an intake staff meeting where all disciplines discuss the patient and the various therapies and interventions needed. This interprofessional team functions collaboratively, listening, seeking clarification, and working for not just information exchange but for communication. Once the patient begins treatment, the health care providers continue to work together to maximize patient outcomes.

For example, Mr. Corbin, a patient who has had a left-hemisphere stroke, is receiving therapy from a SLP for expressive aphasia and swallowing; a PT to improve walking and balance; an OT to regain the ability to perform ADLs such as dressing, bathing, and writing; and a dietitian to manage a healthy diet that has been modified for the swallowing problems he is experiencing. As part of IPCP, the team works together to develop an optimal treatment schedule. For example, the SLP noticed

(continued)

Case Study (continued)

that Mr. Corbin could not participate in swallowing exercises without falling asleep. The SLP and the PT coordinated their treatment schedule so that Mr. Corbin did not have PT until after SLP therapy. The PT provided the SLP with techniques for positioning Mr. Corbin to maximize the efficacy of the swallowing exercises. The OT worked with the PT, dietitian, SLP, and nurses to ensure the adaptive dining utensils were available and being used to help develop independent feeding.

Due to an administration-initiated change, the SLP is replaced. The new team member starts adjusting patient treatment schedules to facilitate the efficiency of the SLP schedule across the day. This means that Mr. Corbin's treatment is sometimes scheduled before and sometimes after the PT session. The SLP professional is timely in charting progress and documenting the changes in Mr. Corbin's modified diet required for safe oral feeding, but she also regularly misses team meetings and does not find it necessary to consult with the other health care professionals to ensure the team is aware when changes are made to treatment plans.

Mr. Corbin's case is just one example of the types of issues experienced by the health care team and their patients. Several team members have spoken to you because the team is not functioning well. When the SLP professional walks into the room, other team members stop talking and leave. What are some of the communication problems interfering with patient care? How are team members dealing with the problems they are experiencing?

Communication allows us to connect or to reach others with our wants, needs, and ideas. It is critical to the success of team building and is a phenomenon that drives us all. When we are successful in our communication, a shared understanding develops that helps to secure a desired outcome. Unsuccessful communication can result in frustration, ineffective interactions, and failure to achieve team goals and client outcomes. Many books and articles have been written to address communication within groups and organizations. Research on effective communication notes an increase in complexity when dialogue moves from a single speaker and single listener to small groups. In addition to the number of people involved in the act of communication, IPCP in health care has the added element of communicating for the primary purpose of delivering high-quality client care. In fact, communication is considered one of the most essential components of a successful team,[1-3] and yet effective communication is one of the most challenging dynamics for any group to achieve.

Considering the number and types of professionals who may be part of an interprofessional health care team, it is understandable how communication may get in the way of effective practice. To that end, the purpose of this chapter is to provide a framework for the components of communication and some possible reasons for miscommunications when they occur. Additionally, strategies that can enhance communication within health care teams will be reviewed.

Overview of Team Communication

When thinking about communication within teams, it is important to remember that team members are simultaneously sending and receiving messages.[4] To be understood by others, it is critical that the person sending the message and the person receiving the message share the intended meaning. The speech chain (figure 7.1), as described by Hulit, Fahey, and Howard,[5] can be used to explain the act of communication between individuals.

1. The first step of the speech chain is neurological and takes the form of the ideas the speaker wishes to communicate to the listener. This step occurs quickly and requires a significant amount of cognitive processing. For example, if a colleague asks how you are, it takes only milliseconds to decide if you want to provide a detailed answer or simply reply with, "Fine, how are you?"
2. In the second step, the exact words are selected and arranged in grammatical order. Unless you are consciously making decisions about your word choices, this step is subconscious.
3. The third step happens when your motor cortex is activated and neurological impulses are sent to the appropriate muscles for speech, respiration, and limbs.
4. The fourth step consists of vocal-fold vibration and oral-mechanism movement that result in the acoustic waves known as speech.
5. The fifth step occurs when these acoustic waves reach the listener's eardrum, activating the mechanical processes in the middle ear and subsequently the hydraulic operations in the inner ear.
6. In the sixth and last step, which only takes milliseconds, the signal has navigated the acoustic nerve to the auditory cortex, where the brain detects sound, interprets the sound as speech, and processes it for meaning.

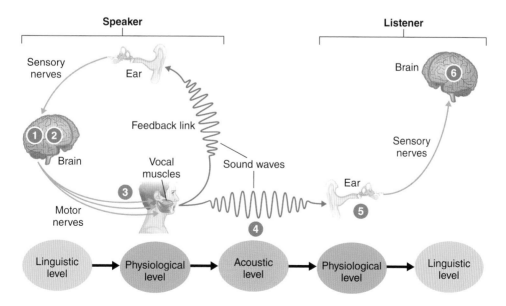

Figure 7.1   Speech chain.

Although the speech chain is a tidy explanation, effective communication only occurs if the person receiving the information understands the message as intended by the person sending it.[1]

Verbal Communication

The speech chain provides a simplistic view of verbal communication consisting of an acoustic signal, words, and sentences spoken out loud. Verbal communication is governed by rules concerning how to put sounds together into words (i.e., phonology), how to put words together into meaningful sentences (i.e., semantics and syntax), and how to put sentences together into larger units of meaning (i.e., discourse). Many cognitive processes are engaged before the acoustic signal, the foundation of an attempt to communicate with a listener, is produced. Language is a cognitive process by which individuals map meaning onto their world, and communication is the attempt to share the meaning created, via internal processes, with others. Ensuring that the speaker and listener understand a shared meaning is essential for the act of communication to occur.

The more abstract the verbal communication, the easier it is to miscommunicate. For example, as a team works together to create a diet that is safe for a patient with a swallowing disorder, the team, including caregivers, will have to create a common meaning of *safe*. The dietitian's definition of *safe* may include the number of calories for the patient to ingest, the physician's definition may be restricted to anything that cannot be aspirated, the family's definition may include the foods the patient will eat, and so on. Team communication for the purpose of problem solving and resourcefulness in health care involves an abundance of words with ambiguous meaning and variations in meaning among health care providers and disciplines. Bypassing occurs when interprofessional team members assume that everyone understands what is being said. The lack of perspective taking, indicative of bypassing, can be a source of misunderstandings and confusions among the members of the interprofessional team and the cause of inefficient and ineffective patient care.[6]

Verbal communication consists of sharing meaning via the spoken or written language channel. It relies on an acoustic signal or written language made up of speech sounds that are arranged into words and sentences, all of which carry meaning. When patient care is at stake, it is imperative that interprofessional team members work to establish shared meaning. To provide quality patient care, communicating results, accommodations, treatment plans, and so on, it is critical that all team members ensure they understand the ideas being presented.

Speaking sentences and establishing shared meaning are an important part of communicating ideas, but they only account for a portion of the act of communicating. A significant part of understanding a verbal message is the information carried by nonverbal communication.

Nonverbal Communication

Nonverbal communication is defined by Borkowski "as sharing information without using words to encode messages"[1(p87)] and is an important part of the communication process. At its most basic, nonverbal communication can be understood even if the speaker is nonverbal or speaks a different language. Communicative gestures carry meaning, and we use them before we develop oral language and maintain them after we lose the ability to use oral language. Examples of easy-to-understand nonverbal communication include a person with expressive aphasia pointing at something she wants, putting her hand up as a form of rejection, or nodding her head in agreement. Nonverbal language can be complicated and may indicate that the meaning expressed using oral language is actually the opposite of the intended meaning, as is the case with sarcasm.

According to Nelson and Quick,[7] there are 4 components of nonverbal communication:

1. **Proxemics** is concerned with the use of space for communication. Examples of proxemics can be the seating arrangements for meetings or how close someone stands when talking to another person.

2. **Kinesthetics** consists of using body language and gestures to communicate messages. Body language and gestures can signal a closed or open communication style. For example, crossed arms during a meeting convey that a team member is closed off to the discussion. Other types of body language that can indicate closed communication include crossing legs when seating or standing and tapping or drumming fingers.

3. **Facial expression and eye behavior** tell the emotional state of both listeners and speakers.

4. **Paralinguistics** (i.e., suprasegmental or prosodic features) include the speaker's pitch, volume, and junctures. Listeners use paralinguistic features to identify syllable stress and word, phrase, and sentence boundaries of connected speech. For example, paralinguistic features mark or emphasize essential words or phrases and differentiate word meaning and function (e.g., the noun *CON-tract* versus the verb *con-TRACT*). Humor and some forms of nonliteral language, such as sarcasm and irony, rely heavily on paralinguistic features to ensure the intent is communicated.

A significant amount of information is communicated nonverbally. In fact, Mehrabian[8] suggests that only 7% of the speaker's message is communicated by the words used. Communicative intent is interpreted using both verbal and nonverbal signals, and as health care teams interact, members must remember that nonverbal communication is the more powerful tool when sending and receiving messages.

TOOLS OF IPE
Tips for Improving Nonverbal Communication

Many times miscommunications happen not because of what we do intentionally but because of what we do unintentionally. When interacting with other team members either in didactic or group communication, remember that 93% of what you communicate is nonverbal.

- Choose body language that is open by leaning your head to one side, keeping your arms down, and standing with your shoulders back.
- Be conscious about eye contact, keeping in mind that uninterrupted eye contact is considered intimidating.
- Acknowledge agreement with the speaker by smiling or slightly nodding your head.
- Devices such as sarcasm are best left out of the workplace; they are easily misunderstood.
- Lean in when someone is talking to you in order to indicate interest.

Small-Group Communication

As health care teams work toward the common goal of patient care, they will use a variety of communication venues (e.g., written, oral, virtual), all of which have one thing in common: a sender and a receiver. Awareness that these factors can cause misunderstandings does not mean no miscommunications will occur. However, an understanding that different people have different cultures, may speak in a variety of dialects, and use gender-specific communication styles can enable the interprofessional team to work through misunderstandings, keeping in mind that the goal is to provide quality patient care.

Chandler[9] suggests that making meaning from a conversation is an active process whereby the listener creates meaning based not only on the information presented but also on the listener's internal lexicon, past experiences, and biases. Programs that educate health care professionals teach the communication skills necessary for didactic, or one-on-one, communication. Techniques such as asking open-ended questions, limiting professional jargon, using active listening, and having caring intent are usually taught in educational programs and have been identified as essential elements of didactic interpersonal communication skills for health care professionals.[6,10]

Small-group, or team, interaction requires additional communication skills with various factors, such as managing power differentials and clarity of messages, that can influence the team's success. Any team member's message has the potential for misunderstanding, which increases exponentially with each additional group member. The more listeners involved in trying to understand the speaker, the greater the variety of understandings that can occur. When speaking to a group, the possibility for miscommunication increases logarithmically. Lake and colleagues[6] describe the potential for miscommunications in this way: When person A is talking to person B, the active meaning-making process has a direct path from A to B. When you have 4 people in a group, with A being the speaker and then B, C, and D being the listeners, communication becomes multidirectional (AB, AC, AD, BC, BD, and CD). Duffy and colleagues[10] found that small-group communication, although necessary for successful interprofessional team interaction, is not explicitly taught to health care professionals as frequently as didactic communication.

Klinzing and Klinzing[11] identify 3 areas of potential areas of communication breakdowns in group communication.

1. *Factual or inference confusion*—Factual statements using language that is observable can reduce the risk of misunderstanding. Statements such as "The patient participated in therapy for 10 minutes and then requested a break" use observable language that leaves little room for inference. An inferential statement such as "The patient was uncooperative," on the other hand, is more subjective and difficult to observe. The speaker's tone may also influence the listener's interpretation, giving an inferential statement the weight of fact.

2. *Overgeneralization*—Superordinate nouns (e.g., *foreigners, doctors, alcoholics*), nonspecific verbs (e.g., *use, go, is, can*), and qualifiers (e.g., *always, all, very, never*) can preserve stereotypes and overgeneralization. An example of an overgeneralized statement would be something like, "PTs always work on gross motor and OTs work on fine motor." This statement includes superordinate nouns, *PTs* and *OTs*, and a qualifier, *always*.

3. *Polarizing language*—The use of either–or language (e.g., good or bad, compliant or uncompliant) can promote black-and-white thinking and oversimplify circumstances. Taking the time to engage in thoughtful communication can eliminate these types of problems.

Reducing qualifiers and polarizing language by being careful with word choices and introducing inferences with I-statements is important for precise and efficient communication.

Interprofessional Communication

Although there is no one formula for effective communication, IPEC[12] developed an extensive set of communication competencies that provide a framework to help interprofessional teams develop the skills necessary to provide efficient and effective communication. The first competency requires that the team "choose effective communication tools and techniques, including information systems and communication technologies, to facilitate discussions and interactions that enhance team function."[12(p23)] Another competency requires the team "use respectful language appropriate for a given difficult situation, crucial conversation, or interprofessional conflict."[12(p23)] There are 8 specific competencies that include foundational skills areas such as avoiding jargon, providing constructive feedback when needed, avoiding professional bias, and engaging in active listening (see the IPEC Effective Verbal Communication Competencies sidebar for the complete list).

EBP OF TEAMSHIP
Communication Styles of Two Teams

Sheehan, Robertson, and Ormond (2007) compared the communication styles of interprofessional teams versus multidisciplinary teams to better understand the influence of the philosophical underpinnings on communication and role understanding. These authors used a symbolic interactionist approach for the purpose of identifying communication patterns. Using the interview data, they analyzed the language used by team members during and after patient discharge from treatment. The interprofessional team members' language was characterized by shared linguistic practices that included consistency of terminology and common understanding of goals, decision making as a team, and valuing team members. In contrast, the multidisciplinary team members' use of language provided less evidence of working collaboratively and respect for team member roles and more individual decision making. The authors concluded that working on an interprofessional team involves a more astute awareness of social interaction within the team, resulting in role sharing and collaboration.[27]

TOOLS OF IPE
IPEC Effective Verbal Communication Competencies

Because communication is critical for interprofessional health care teams to function effectively and efficiently, IPEC identified the following competencies for communication:[12]

- Select effective communication tools and techniques to enhance team functions.
- Use language that is easy to understand when communicating with others about patient care.
- Be respectful, clear, and confident when communicating health care information and having difficult interprofessional team conversations.
- Use active listening techniques and nonverbal communication to encourage an open exchange of ideas.
- Provide timely and constructive feedback to other interprofessional team members.
- Use respectful language, keeping in mind the difficulty of the situation or possible conflict.
- Be aware of how your background, experiences, influence, and authority contribute positively or negatively to the efficiency of an interprofessional team.
- Advocate the importance of teamwork in health care situations.

Individual Differences

Interprofessional teams are by definition composed of people from different disciplines, and each member brings to the table a variety of best practices, scopes of practice, and territorial issues. For an interprofessional team to be functional, the group must navigate these issues to develop collaborative strategies that hold paramount the patient's welfare. Another layer of individuality that can cause difficulty is the fact that team members all bring their personal or cultural experiences, and they may or may not share the same dialect or native language. Additionally, the team is likely to consist of members with different genders or who identify as gender neutral. If not managed, these and other individual differences can affect the interprofessional team's ability to communicate and subsequently provide quality patient care.

The interpretation of a spoken or written message is influenced by a listener's culturally influenced life experiences. The sensitivity and care with which an interprofessional team handles cultural differences can have an impact on its success. Many cultures make up the United States. Cultural identity can include geographical parameters, such as southern or northern, and it can be based on ethnicity, race, or group affiliation. These and other mechanisms for defining a person's culture are equally valid, if perhaps a little simplistic.

Another way to discuss cultural differences is with the notion of high-context and low-context cultures.[13]

- High-context cultures rely heavily on nonverbal communication with a focus on relationship building. Because relationships are important, disagreements may become personalized.

- Low-context cultures tend to rely on written communication, with rule-governed interactions and data-driven decision making.

It is not surprising that interactions may be riddled with miscommunications when a team has members from high-context and low-context cultures. Unless interprofessional teams are aware of these types of cultural differences, people from high-context cultures may take disagreements personally while those from low-context cultures may be clueless about what went wrong.

When team members come from culturally and linguistically diverse backgrounds, communication difficulties can also occur because of language differences. An easy way to tell if you are having a conversation with people who use a different dialect than you is to listen to how they say their words. They might use different vowels to pronounce *pen* and *pin*, or they might use different words for common objects, such as calling carbonated beverages *soda* and not *pop*. Even though there are more than 20 regional dialects in the United States, (e.g., Ozark, Southern Appalachian, Hudson Valley, Southwestern),[14] dialects are mutually intelligible versions of a language, so by definition speakers should be able to understand the words that are being said. However, Taylor's[15] definition of dialects may better describe the nature of culture as a multifaceted interaction of a group's shared history, which includes cultural, educational, social, and linguistic influences. Taylor's definition highlights the fact that dialect can be tied to identity and should be managed with thoughtfulness and sensitivity.

Gender Differences

Differences in communication style between men and women have been well documented, along with difficulties these differences can cause in the workplace,[16,17] and include characteristics such as women making more eye contact and facing their partner more than men. Men tend to interrupt the speaker more and are more likely to share their accomplishments than women. Men generally make more declarative statements, such as "The patient must see the OT before breakfast," whereas women use more qualifiers, such as "Maybe we should schedule OT treatment for the patient before breakfast." These examples are not valid for all men or all women, but they are some examples of gender-specific speaking styles that may cause misunderstandings when teams include both men and women.

Professional Arrogance

Another communication-related topic to address is the professional bias, or professional arrogance, that can occur when two or more health care professionals interact for patient care. The notion of professional arrogance comes from the nature of a professional, which is someone who has engaged in an activity that requires intense study to master. Burch[18] suggests that how students learn a discipline's scope of practice within a domain-specific body of literature creates an exclusivity, or territorialism, that hinders the formation of interprofessional relationships. Burch[18] and McNair[19] both suggest that a fundamental way to fight professional bias is to provide students with regular IPE opportunities that reinforce foundational principles of patient care above professional tribalism. Additionally, health care teams may find it necessary to strategically and intentionally engage in a variety of communication strategies (see the next section) to minimize the effects of professional arrogance.

General Communication Strategies

The goal of interprofessional teams is to offer patients effective and efficient treatment, and communication is a factor that influences the ability to meet that goal. Klinzing and Klinzing[11] have identified some internal and external forces that interfere with the ability to engage in conversations or meetings:

- The mind processes words faster than they can be spoken, which can result in the formulation of responses before the message has been delivered.
- As people try to multitask, they experience divided attention, which can interfere with the ability to sustain attention during meetings.
- Environmental distractors, such as cell phones, noise in the hall, and shuffling feet, can interrupt attention.

If we allow things to compete for our attention when we are in a meeting, then we stop being communication collaborators.

Communication is a complex process, and both speakers and listeners carry responsibility for success. We have identified 9 actions (modified from Seery)[20] that can support interprofessional teams in their communication efforts.

1. Use Engaged Listening

We have all experienced talking to people and knowing they were not listening. The listeners may be physically distracted, checking their watch or looking at their phone. They may appear distracted, and it is evident they are thinking about something other than what you are saying.

Engaged listening is required for effective communication, and it involves actually hearing and trying to understand what the speaker intends for you to understand. When listening, you can gain clarification by asking questions or rephrasing what you are hearing so that you're sure you fully understand the message as intended. Lake and her colleagues[6] remind us that listeners share responsibility for ensuring they have an accurate and complete understanding of the message. They suggest the following techniques for active listening:

- Resolve differences between verbal and nonverbal messages.
- Reflect your feelings about what is being said.
- Ask clarification questions.
- Restate the speaker's message.

Using these techniques helps make communication a process that is a partnership between speaker and listener.

2. Use Nonverbal Communication

As stated previously, the words we select for the sentences we say make up only 7% of the message being conveyed. For both speaker and listener, the conscious use of proxemics, kinesthetics, facial expression and eye behavior, and paralinguistics can reduce miscommunications. For example, your body language should help convey your words and should indicate your openness to the message being sent. Other nonverbal communication acts, such as standing or sitting (proxemics), hand gestures (kinesthetics), eye contact (facial expression and eye behavior), and voice tone (paralinguistics), can enhance communication. For example, a team member may be more likely to speak openly if you are relaxed, have a friendly tone, and use an open posture with uncrossed legs and arms. Eye contact is also important; too much can be intimidating and too little can indicate you are nervous or disengaged. Conscious use of nonverbal cues can help counteract some of the professional, cultural, and linguistic differences you are likely to encounter on interprofessional teams. You can also use your understanding of nonverbal cues to interpret how other team members are feeling.

3. Be Concise and Clear

Team members' time is important, so you should be as concise as possible. Understanding the purpose of your interaction can help you stay focused and convey only the relevant information, which in turn helps the team achieve its common goal efficiently. You should not sacrifice clarity for conciseness, however. Be mindful of shared meaning; group diversity (e.g., professional, cultural, dialectical) could make jargon, professional acronyms, and colloquialisms problematic. Failure to be both concise and clear can cause frustration and confusion.

4. Be Personable

Everyone likes to work with someone who is pleasant, agreeable, and kind. These are some of the characteristics that could be considered personable. Using both verbal and nonverbal communication can help convey information about yourself. This can be as simple as smiling and nodding when you agree with what is being said, managing your tone so that passion does not sound like aggression, allowing others to state their opinion first so that you appear receptive to other ideas, or adding a personal message to an email so that your communication is less abrupt.

5. Speak With Confidence

When you convey to other team members that you are up to the task, then effective communication can occur. If you sound tentative about your contribution to the team, the team will be cautious about your ability to help meet the goal. Using nonverbal cues such as tone and stance can help portray confidence. You should also listen to the message others are communicating and then use engaged listening to seek clarification.

6. Show Empathy

Empathy, the ability to take the perspective of another person or to understand what someone is feeling, is a foundational skill for successful interactions. You do not have to agree with what people are saying to show that you appreciate their perspective. By saying to your team members, "I understand where you are coming from," you let them know that you have heard their message. Remember that people from low-context and high-context cultures will react differently to disagreements, so use other tools to ensure relationships among group members stay intact.

7. Stay Open-Minded

We have discussed cultural, dialectical, and gender differences, all of which can influence shared meaning, relationships, and decision making. Using all of your tools to project openness to others' opinions and ideas is necessary for honest and effective communication.

8. Give and Receive Feedback

When you ask for clarification or restate something that has been said, you are providing feedback about your understanding and potentially about the effectiveness of the interaction. This is an essential skill for communication and for the interprofessional team to be efficient and effective. There are other types of devices as well, such as praising someone's presentation or providing supportive, constructive feedback that can strengthen any team. How you give and receive feedback can affect team morale, so having a handle on the cultural differences within the group can help you frame your questions and feedback.

EBP OF TEAMSHIP
Closed-Loop Communication

Closed-loop communication (CLC) is a well-known team communication technique that has been studied as a mechanism for providing feedback in health care settings when performing collaborative tasks. It is often used during medical procedures and is adaptable for other health care teams. CLC consists of 3 steps:

1. A team member calls out an observation or message.
2. The second team member confirms that the message was received.
3. The first team member confirms that original message was understood correctly.

For example, during a team meeting, a nurse states that the patient is NPO. The PT on the team confirms that the patient cannot be given any food or liquids by mouth. The nurse confirms by stating, "That is correct, the patient cannot be given any food or drink even if the patient requests it."

In a case study, Johnson and colleagues[21] investigated CLC along with two other communication techniques, shared mental model (SMM) and mutual trust (MT). SMM is based on the notion that, over time, team members develop a common context that facilitates understanding and the prediction of outcomes. MT is based on the shared belief that team members will do what they are supposed to do and that their actions will protect the team. The authors found that CLC was most helpful to team communication when used in conjunction with SMM.

9. Consider the Medium

A large part of figuring out the medium (e.g., oral, written, electronic) for any communication is considering the audience and purpose. Remember, when contemplating a written format, only a small portion of any attempt to communicate is conveyed by the words selected. Sensitive information may best be handled in person. Some communication devices, such as humor and sarcasm, use paralinguistic features and can fall flat when using written language. Additionally, when selecting a communication medium, careful thought should be given to any content that is sensitive or confidential.

Lake and colleagues[6] suggest that structured reflection is useful to monitor and increase self-awareness as you practice communication techniques within your interprofessional team. Self-reflection can take the form of journaling and checklists

COLLABORATIVE CORNER
Self-Reflection

You may want to start your self-reflection with the following types of questions:

- What message am I sending?
- Who am I trying to convince and why?
- Is the purpose of my communication to achieve a group goal or a personal one?
- Am I open to the other ideas presented?
- How do I want my message received, or how was my message received?

before or after meetings and interactions. Choosing good communication strategies, consciously using them in conversations and meetings, and evaluating both your successes and failures is important for your individual success as well as for doing your part to ensure that the interprofessional team is effective and efficient.

Specific Communication Strategies

Because teamwork is not easy and requires a willingness to build relationships, develop personal communication skills, and work toward consensus and compromise, many specific strategies have been designed to facilitate interprofessional team communication. Most put a more structured framework on the general communication strategies, which can make the strategies easier for interprofessional teams to use. Typically, a workplace or an interprofessional team will make an intentional decision and select a specific strategy to use.

LAFF, Don't CRY

McNaughton and Vostal[22] developed a communication technique called *LAFF, don't CRY* to encourage active learning in teams. With this strategy, team members should avoid the following:

- **C**riticizing people who are not present
- **R**eacting quickly or making a promise that cannot be kept
- **Y**akking or going on about a personal experience, causing the group to lose sight of the goal

Instead, team members should do the following:

- **L**isten, empathize, and communicate respect.
- **A**sk questions and permission to take meeting notes.
- **F**ocus on the issues.
- **F**ind a first step or goal.

This technique can support communication within the interprofessional health care team by encouraging active listening and goal-directed behavior. It can stop unproductive complaining and create a situation where the team is working toward a resolution. The notion of ending the meeting with a goal, even if the goal is to gather additional information and meet again on a specific date, creates forward movement and team progress.

SBAR

SBAR (situation, background, assessment, and recommendation) is another strategy that provides a template for communicating information within a clinical environment. It's a great strategy to help health care teams develop clear and concise communication. For example, this technique can be applied when the health care team is staffing patients during intake. Before beginning your communication, you should have conducted a thorough chart review and assessment.

- *Situation*—State your name, position, work setting, topic, and the time needed to discuss.
- *Background*—State the problem or patient diagnosis and pertinent medical information.
- *Assessment*—Present assessment results.
- *Recommendation*—Present the treatment plan.

SBAR is rather straightforward and can be used in both group (e.g., grand rounds, shift changes) and didactic interactions.[23]

CORBS

Another method for effective interprofessional team communication feedback is CORBS (clear, owned, regular, balanced, and specific), as described by Hawkins and Shohet.[24] This strategy for interaction has been used in health care settings to structure feedback.

- *Clear*—Use clear and concise language to communicate your point. Being vague is frustrating to the listener and not effective or efficient.
- *Owned*—Your feedback is based on your perceptions, and it belongs to you. You should use I-statements (e.g., "I notice in your presentation . . .").
- *Regular*—Provide feedback often and as soon as possible.
- *Balanced*—Do not focus on negative feedback, although you do not have to counterbalance negative feedback with positive.
- *Specific*—Use language that is specific and observable.

CORBS has been demonstrated to be useful in training situations[25] and could be employed in interprofessional team interactions where feedback is part of the communication process. This strategy incorporates many of the IPEC competencies for effective verbal communication[12] described earlier in the chapter.

Electronic Health Records and Team Communication

Electronic health records (EHR) have changed the landscape of interprofessional team communication, taking it from face-to-face debriefing or reading a paper medical chart to a ubiquitous electronic experience. Although there is some early evidence that EHR can enhance IPCP and communication, Rashotte and colleagues[26] suggest that more longitudinal evidence should be gathered to determine its impact on patient outcomes.

Included on any interprofessional team are the patients and caregivers, who may need help developing communication strategies to fully participate in their own health care. Programs such as the Speak Up campaign from the Joint Commission and phone and computer application for patient access to EHR can facilitate communication with the health care team. These strategies provide interprofessional teams with explicit steps that can aid in interactions that enhance patient care.

TOOLS OF IPE
Speak Up Campaign

The Speak Up campaign was developed to encourage patients to speak up about their own care. It offers an extensive library with materials that include videos (in English and Spanish), infographics, handouts, and artwork. Following are some of the topics:

- Infection control
- Antibiotics
- X-rays and MRIs
- Depression
- Falling risk
- Surgical errors
- Memory problems and dementia
- Stroke

These materials are available to download by performing an Internet search using the phrase "Speak Up campaign."

Summary

There is no one way to ensure that what you want to communicate has been understood as intended, and there are many factors that can interfere with conveying your ideas. The complex nature of shared meaning and the multitude of factors, internal and external, that can disrupt communication can be detrimental to the ability of an interprofessional team to provide the most efficient and effective patient care. Understanding the components of communication and interprofessional teams' verbal and nonverbal communication, group diversity, and group communication can illuminate areas where breakdowns can occur.

Using both general and specific strategies for communication can help interprofessional teams develop the skills needed to interact effectively. If the team practices these strategies, then when misunderstandings occur—and they will occur—the team has created a climate conducive to effective and efficient communication. Evidence-based communication strategies, such as SBAR and CORBS, provide teams with proven methods to improve patient care. A team using effective communication will undoubtedly produce positive collaborative interactions that benefit the patient. In chapter 8, we will review how IPE and ICPC initiatives can move from project-based to sustainable practices.

CASE STUDY Debriefing

Communication among interprofessional team members is essential for the effective and efficient treatment of patients. Before the personnel change at the rehabilitation center, the health care providers were functioning as a team. They had regular meetings and coordinated treatment plans. They worked out problems with scheduling, making adjustments that were for the good of the patient. This is how interprofessional teams should function—pulling together for the patient. Then the environment changed and the team was no longer functional.

It would be easy to blame the SLP for not being a team player by not joining staff meetings, expecting the other team members to know when she updated her patient's treatment plans in the medical charts, and putting her schedule above those of the other team members, including Mr. Corbin. We have learned that there are communication strategies that can improve team function, and it appears that the SLP, a communication specialist by the way, did not employ any of them. If you will remember, 93% of communication is conveyed nonverbally, and the SLP's lack of engagement may very well have been communicating her disinterest in being part of the team.

But there is another lens from which to view this scenario, and it will lay blame for the breakdown in communication on the existing members of the team. When team members engage in good communication practices, they are explicit in their use and help each other by selecting effective communication techniques. They also provide timely and productive feedback to other team members. Additionally, they advocate the importance of teamwork in health care situations. Interprofessional health care teams require both didactic and group communication and intentional use of communication strategies to ensure understanding.

(continued)

Case Study *(continued)*

Case Study Discussion Questions

1. Discuss other factors that could have been influencing the new SLP's lack of engagement.
2. How could the team use some general communication strategies to communicate their expectations to the new member?
3. Discuss some techniques and strategies that the team members could use to increase their communication effectiveness and to prevent this from happening with the next personnel change.

CHAPTER 8

Building Sustainability

Tina Patel Gunaldo, PhD, DPT, MHS
Pamela Waynick-Rogers, DNP, APRN-BC

Objectives

After reading this chapter, the reader will be able to do the following:

- Describe the 3 key elements of a sustainable model.
- Discuss similarities and differences between IPE and IPCP enablers and barriers in academic and practice settings.
- Provide examples of IPCP for the attributes of affordability, acceptability, and adaptability.

CASE STUDY   Sustaining IPCP

Gold Health Care System provides services to the Medicare population through an accountable care organization (ACO). A foundational tenet of ACOs is the development of a coordinated care model.[1] Coordination among providers and hospitals helps to provide high-quality care (i.e., safe, timely, effective, efficient, equitable, and patient-centered care). As members of an administrative team review quality care reports from the past 3 years, they recognize inconsistencies in patient-perception outcome measures where they would like to see consistent service. Specifically, scores relating to respect, courtesy, and listening on the Consumer Assessment of Healthcare Providers and Systems (CAHPS) are inconsistent between professions. Over the past 3 years, individuals trained in reviewing processes, defects, and waste have been integral team members in improving outcomes related to coordinated care, so the administrators consult with the specialized quality team.

During the meeting, it is recognized that the developed processes are fully integrated and systematically occurring. The administrators ask for further investigation and for the patient care teams to reconvene to review the outcomes. The QI team meets with the frontline providers to request further review of the patient perception surveys. Throughout the meeting, the quality team notices potential conflicts among individuals as related to patient care. After the meeting, one of the providers, a recent graduate, approaches the QI team about the lack of IPCP among team members. After the meeting, the quality team reports to the administration that the

(continued)

Case Study *(continued)*

procedures are implemented successfully, but there is a potential conflict among members of the patient care team related to the lack of interprofessional behaviors.

In an effort to address the underlying cause of the conflict, an experienced consultant in IPE and IPCP is hired to evaluate the patient care team. The consultant's report indicates the following:

- A lack of collaboration and communication among team members
- A lack of role clarity and responsibilities
- The possibility that these behavioral observations could be contributing to a plateau of outcome measures

Gold Health Care System leaders decide to address the report and invite the consultant to provide an educational session on IPCP to one of the health provider teams. The attendees evaluate the educational session and make positive remarks about the new information, but they are unsure how to further develop interprofessional behaviors without training and guidance. The administrators support an IPCP environment but need to create a comprehensive plan on how to develop, integrate, and assess collaboration within the health care system and its impact on patient outcomes.

Gold Health Care System leaders decide to build a stronger relationship with neighboring health care educational institutions to increase understanding of IPE and its translation to IPCP. The organization is committed to supporting clinicians in their desire to learn more about an interprofessional approach to the delivery of health care.

The opening case study highlights the widening gap occurring between IPE and IPCP. Chapters 1 through 4 outline the history and need for IPE while providing growing evidence in IPE development, implementation, and assessment. Chapters 5 through 7 discuss the evidence that exists within interprofessional competencies. IPE research is growing at a faster rate than IPCP. Minimizing the gap between IPE in academic programs and IPCP among providers will help build sustainability for the relatively new practice of working in interprofessional teams.

Many initiatives within health care focus on improving quality of care, such as IPE and IPCP. Technology advancements such as EHRs and electronic wearables are examples of products the industry adopts and integrates into daily practice. These pieces of technology can be easier to integrate because of their physical properties. Service-oriented products such as IPCP, on the other hand, challenge the health care system because it is difficult to develop processes and measure outcomes based on nontangible products.

Previous chapters provided foundational aspects of IPCP demonstrating teamwork and interprofessional communication as a science. As research in IPE and IPCP continues to grow and practices are integrated in academic and practice environments, a sustainability model becomes vital in the quest to improve health outcomes. This chapter identifies IPE and IPCP initiatives related to a 3-factor sustainable development model.

Sustainability Factors

The origin of a sustainable development model is linked to the environment and natural resources sector. In the United Nations' *Report of the World Commission on Environment and Development*, *sustainability* is defined as "development that meets the needs of the present without compromising the ability of future generations to meet their own."[2 (p154)] Most noted in the literature are the 3 pillars of sustainability: environment, social, and economic.[3] Sustainability exists where these pillars intersect (figure 8.1).[3] Since the 1980s, the model has been adopted by other industries, such as business, nonprofit organizations, and health care. However, the literature offers minimal discussion on sustainable models and is void of information on IPCP sustainability.

In 2012, Fineberg noted that a sustainable health system has "three key attributes: affordability, for patients and families, employers, and the government (recognizing that employers and the government ultimately rely on individuals as consumers, employees, and taxpayers for their resources); acceptability to key constituents, including patients and health professionals; and adaptability, because health and health care needs are not static (i.e., a health system must respond adaptively to new diseases, changing demographics, scientific discoveries, and dynamic technologies in order to remain viable)."[4(p1020)] The global sustainable model with 3 pillars[3] is analogous to the 3 attributes for a sustainable health system.[4] Affordability is reflective of the economy, and acceptability and adaptability are reflective of society and the environment, respectively (figure 8.2). This chapter will use the terminology in figure 8.2 to outline examples and interactions of each attribute as we investigate the initial attempts to develop sustainable IPE and IPCP models.

The need for IPE and IPCP has been outlined in previous chapters. Proponents of enhanced collaborative efforts in the health care industry cite the prevalence of medical errors,

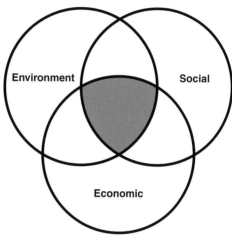

Figure 8.1 Sustainability model.

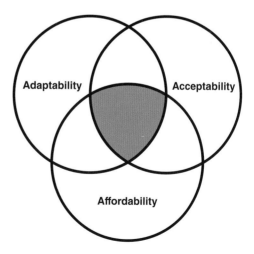

Figure 8.2 Sustainability model for the health care system.

fragmented care, poor health outcomes, and exponential costs associated with health care delivery. There is growing support from the academic, clinical, and community environments for IPE and IPCP, but there is a gap in knowledge gained through IPE research and IPCP practice adoption, as well as a gap in how IPE is delivered based on IPCP research.

Most are familiar with the lag in translating knowledge into action in the health care industry.[5] Balas and Boren report that it takes approximately 17 years for 14% of new research to be adopted.[6] Slow, fragmented adoption of IPCP is a barrier to the delivery of interprofessional care, which has promised to improve quality of care and health outcomes at more affordable costs. In addition, the slow adoption of IPCP is a barrier to developing more meaningful educational models for future health professionals and providers. The knowledge-to-practice gap, as described by Balas and Boren, affects all 3 elements of IPCP sustainability. Therefore, it is critical to incorporate sustainability discussions when designing a new model of education, such as IPE, and delivery to improve health outcomes. IPE and IPCP sustainability and the associated benefits will hinge on narrowing the bidirectional knowledge-to-practice gap in time and percentage of practice adoption.

Lawlis and colleagues coordinated IPE research outcomes related to sustainability, but organized the results related to 3 primary stakeholders: government and professional, institutional, and individual.[7] For each stakeholder, the authors included enablers and barriers for IPE within an academic environment (see the sidebar IPE Enablers and Barriers for Primary Stakeholders). A comparison among the stakeholders indicated that funding, faculty development programs, organizational structures, and individual commitment are key components of sustainability. This comprehensive list was an initial attempt to organize existing research to guide future IPE implementation.

TOOLS OF IPE
Addressing the Knowledge-to-Practice Gap

When prioritizing IPCP at an institution or within a private practice, reflect on how your team can improve these facts: It takes 17 years for research to reach practice, 14% of research reaches a patient, and 18% of administrators and practitioners report using evidence-based practice frequently.[6]

- How can we improve the time it takes for research in IPE to reach clinical practice?
- How can we increase the integration of evidence-based IPCP into patient care?
- How can we coordinate research between academic and clinical practice settings for efficient bidirectional learning?

IPE ENABLERS AND BARRIERS FOR PRIMARY STAKEHOLDERS

Government and Professional

Enablers

- Establishment of collaborative groups from various higher education institutions and organizations
- Stakeholder commitment
- Shared ownership and unified goals
- Government funding

Barriers

- Lack of financial resources
- Changes within the organizations and educational institutions involved

Institution

Enablers

- Funding by institutions
- Development of organizational structures
- Faculty development programs

Barriers

- Lack of financial resources
- Lack of support
- Limited faculty development initiatives
- Scheduling of IPE within current programs
- Different degree calendars (different lengths of degree years for different professions)
- Different degree timetables
- Rigid or condensed curricula
- Extracurricular versus required courses
- Differences in assessment requirements

Individual

Enablers

- Facilitator skills and enthusiasm
- Facilitators and staff as role models

(continued)

IPE Enablers and Barriers for Primary Stakeholders *(continued)*

- Champions of IPE
- Commitment to IPE
- Understanding of IPE and IPCP
- Shared interprofessional vision
- Equal status of team members regardless of position or background

Barriers

- Faculty attitudes
- Lack of rewards for faculty
- High workloads (including teaching and administration)
- Lack of knowledge about other health professions
- Poor understanding of IPE
- Lack of perceived value of IPE
- Different student learning styles
- Turf or professional battles
- Bias toward own profession
- Lack of respect toward other health professions

Reprinted by permission from T.R. Lawlis, J. Anson, and D. Greenfield, "Barriers and Enablers That Influence Sustainable Interprofessional Education: A Literature Review," *Journal of Interprofessional Care* 2014;28, no. 4 (2014): 305-310.

The enablers and barriers noted in the sidebar encompass all 3 dimensions of a sustainable model. The remainder of the chapter will provide additional examples of supportive organizations and systems in each of the pillars. Community and clinical practice organizations should reference the research by Lawlis and colleagues[7] as they develop an IPCP sustainable model using Fineberg's structure of adaptability, acceptability, and affordability.[4] As practice settings develop and implement IPCP, outcomes associated with health, costs, and patient satisfaction should also be measured. As the health industry increases engagement in IPCP research, practice outcomes can guide academic institutions as they refine IPE experiences. Together, the various stakeholders can increase the transfer of knowledge related to IPE and IPCP, ultimately decreasing the knowledge-to-practice gap.

Adaptability (Environment)

A discussion of sustainability models should involve adaptability, including both internal and external organizational environments. Similar to the strengths, weaknesses, opportunities, and threats (SWOT) model for strategic planning, a sustainability model must consider the potential impact of elements internal and external to the organization. Stakeholders engaged in IPCP must define the physical resources, which indirectly and directly influence the sustainability of IPCP initiatives.

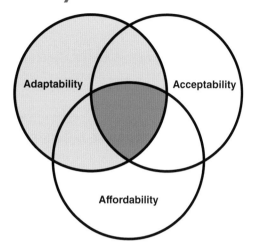

Internal Elements

One of the burning questions asked within the IPE and IPCP community is what influences IPCP. The academic community knows it must prepare future health professionals to demonstrate interprofessional behaviors in clinical practice. However, health care organizations must build upon the current research, which provides initial findings of enablers and barriers to IPCP. Determining these factors will support future IPE and IPCP development. Pullon and colleagues noted 5 key elements affecting IPCP practice:

1. Physical space and layout
2. Location and demographics
3. Business and employment models
4. Shared mission and goals
5. Team structure and climate[9]

Shared areas with adequate space within the clinical environment supported informal communication between health professionals. However, shared areas with limited spaces limited conversation. For example, open doors to offices encouraged discussions, and narrow hallways and small employee break rooms limited conversation.[9]

External Elements

Regarding IPE and IPCP, there is an enormous amount of support from external stakeholders. National and international reports justifying team-based care, educational standards, journals disseminating research, and establishment of a national center can all support individual organizations in their efforts to integrate team-based education and practice.

Academic Institutions

Academic stakeholders, including accrediting organizations, universities, colleges, and programs, have been challenged by WHO and NAM (formerly IOM[10]) to educate students and health professionals in teams. Several national and international reports have advocated for IPE. Specifically, in 1972, a NAM report, *Educating for the Health Team*, recommended instructing students about the various roles, knowledge, and skills of other health professions.[11] More recently, in 2010 WHO reported that IPE is an essential component of IPCP.[12]

Over the past several years, more academic accrediting organizations have written accreditation standards requiring IPE. In 2014, HPAC (Health Professions Accreditors Collaborative) was established to address common areas of interest, including IPE.[13] Today, there are 23 HPAC members.[14] Academic partners are foundational stakeholders in educating future health professionals to be collaborative-practice ready. Chapter 3 provides specific IPE accreditation standards from several health professional programs.

To minimize the knowledge-to-practice gap between current students and health professionals, academic institutions have developed graduate-level degrees focused on IPE. As previously noted, IPE training should occur throughout the career of a health professional. In 2003, NAM challenged the health education system to support the development of teams.[15] Individuals completing graduate programs in IPE will be able to lead in the development of IPCP environments and teams. Currently, Rosalind Franklin University offers a PhD program in Interprofessional Healthcare Studies,[16] and the University of California San Francisco offers a Master of Science program in Healthcare Administration and Interprofessional Leadership.[17]

In addition to a structured curriculum focused on IPE, the United States also supports interprofessional continuing education. In 2009, the Joint Accreditation for Interprofessional Continuing Education was established to support IPE training and decrease administrative burden related to seeking approval to provide continuing education for multiple professions.[18] The Joint Accreditation provides organizations with a single administrative process to apply for approval to provide continuing education for nursing, medicine, optometry, pharmacy, and PA professionals.[18] Organizations who have Joint Accreditation can provide education with a traditional silo focus or IPCP focus[18]; accredited providers can be found on the website.[19]

Supporting Health Organizations

Several organizations support the development, implementation, and assessment of IPE and IPCP. Examples include the Josiah Macy Jr. Foundation, AHRQ (Agency for Healthcare Research and Quality), HRSA (Health Resources and Services Administration), IPEC (Interprofessional Education Collaborative), NAM (National Academy of Medicine), RWJF (Robert Wood Johnson Foundation), and WHO (World Health Organization). The Josiah Macy Jr. Foundation, IPEC, NAM, RWJF, and WHO have published multiple reports highlighting IPE and IPCP. The sidebar on supportive organizations provides a selective list of IPE and IPCP reports.

SUPPORTING ORGANIZATIONS OF IPE AND IPCP AND THEIR RESPECTIVE PUBLICATIONS

Health Professions Accreditors Collaborative (HPAC)
- Guidance on Developing Quality Interprofessional Education for the Health Professions (2019)[38]

Interprofessional Education Collaborative (IPEC)
- Core Competencies for Interprofessional Collaborative Practice (2011 and 2016 Update)[20]

Interprofessional Research Global
- Guidance on Global Interprofessional Education and Collaborative Practice Research: Discussion Paper (2019)[43]

Josiah Macy Jr. Foundation
- Team-Based Competencies: Building a Shared Foundation for Education and Clinical Practice (2011)[21]
- Conference on Interprofessional Education (2012)[21]
- 2012 Annual Report: Accelerating Interprofessional Education[21]
- Conference Summary: Transforming Patient Care: Aligning IPE with Clinical Practice Redesign (2013)[21]
- Transforming Patient Care: Aligning IPE with Clinical Practice Redesign (2013)[21]
- Transforming Patient Care: Aligning Interprofessional Education With Clinical Practice (2013)[21]
- Interprofessional Care Coordination: Looking to the Future (2013)[21]
- Partnering with Patients, Families, and Communities: An Urgent Imperative for Healthcare (2014)[21]
- Partnering with Patients, Families, and Communities to Link Interprofessional Practice and Education (2014)[21]
- 2015 Annual Meeting of the Macy Faculty Scholars[21]

National Academy of Medicine (NAM)
- Core Principles and Values of Effective Team-Based Health Care (2012)[22]
- Interprofessional Education for Collaboration: Learning How to Improve Health From Interprofessional Models Across the Continuum of Education to Practice—Workshop Summary (2013)[23]
- Measuring the Impact of Interprofessional Education (IPE) on Collaborative Practice and Patient Outcomes (2015)[8]
- Strengthening the Connection Between Health Professions Education and Practice: Proceedings of a Joint Workshop (2019)[44]

(continued)

Supporting Organizations of IPE and IPCP and Their Respective
Publications *(continued)*

National Center for Interprofessional Practice and Education
- Guidance on Developing Quality Interprofessional Education for the Health Professions (2019)[38]

National Collaborative for Improving the Clinical Learning Environment (NCICLE)
- Achieving the Optimal Interprofessional Clinical Learning Environment (2019)[39]

Robert Wood Johnson Foundation (RWJF)
- Team-Based Competencies: Building a Shared Foundation for Education and Clinical Practice (2011)[21]
- Lessons from the Field: Promising Interprofessional Collaboration Practices (2015)[24]

The Center for the Advancement of Interprofessional Education (CAIPE)
- Interprofessional Education–The Genesis of Global Movement (2015)[45]
- Interprofessional Education Guidelines (2017)[46]
- CAIPE Fellows Statement on Integrative Care (2017)[47]

World Health Organization (WHO)
- Framework for Action on Interprofessional Education and Collaborative Practice (2010)[12]
- Interprofessional Collaborative Practice in Primary Health Care: Nursing and Midwifery Perspectives (2013)[25]
- Interprofessional Collaborative Practice in Primary Health Care: Nursing and Midwifery Perspectives, Six Case Studies (2013)[26]

In 2012, National Center for Interprofessional Practice and Education was established as the hub for IPE and IPCP. Financial supporters of the National Center include the Josiah Macy Jr. Foundation, Gordon and Betty Moore Foundation, John A. Hartford Foundation, University of Minnesota, HRSA, and RWJF.[27] In addition to supporting IPE from a foundational structure perspective, HRSA also continues to offer grant opportunities that include IPE and IPCP.

AHRQ, a division of HHS, also supports IPCP through the development of Team-STEPPS training modules. TeamSTEPPS are team strategies and tools to enhance performance and patient safety. The TeamSTEPPS delivery system has 3 phases:

- Assess the need
- Plan, train, and implement
- Sustain[28]

During the initial phase, AHRQ advocates for the site to establish a multidisciplinary team dedicated to organizational and cultural change.[28] This recommendation is aligned with IPE enablers noted by Lawlis and colleagues.[7] In addition, sustaining the change will rely on support from administration to incorporate team training as a lifelong learning skill. The support from all of the organizations noted in this section is critical to building a sustainable bridge between IPE and IPCP.

Journals

One source of new knowledge derives from peer-reviewed journals. Currently, there are 4 national and international peer-reviewed interprofessional journals:

1. *Journal of Interprofessional Care*
2. *Health, Interprofessional Practice and Education*
3. *Journal of Interprofessional Education and Practice*
4. *Journal of Research in Interprofessional Practice and Education*

Most of the research published in these journals represents IPE. The fact that interprofessional research is originating from academic institutions is not surprising; many academic health programs have IPE accreditation requirements. Academic accreditation requirements mean that the clinical and community environments can model IPCP training and implementation from the IPE literature. However, recognizing the literature gap between IPE and IPCP and the need to increase IPCP research is critical to sustainability.

Acceptability (Social)

Another component of sustainability is the **acceptability** of IPE in the health care system.[4] Acceptability is not only important for clinicians but for administrators, staff, and patients as well. The importance of buy-in from the various parties cannot be underestimated.[29,30] Patients are particularly essential in this process. Incorporating patient preferences contributes to increased patient engagement and higher-value health care.[31] An additional component of patient engagement is revising accreditation standards to include input from patients, families, and communities.[31]

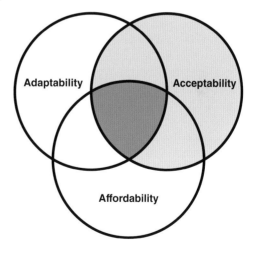

The acceptability of IPE begins while students are in their academic programs in the hopes that the behavior can continue into professional practice.[12] The evidence to support this rationale is discussed in chapter 4. However, this evidence can support how IPE and IPCP are accepted as a normative process in health care. As new clinicians complete their educational programs and IPE and IPCP become a normative process, IPCP is more likely to be supported and encouraged in the clinical setting.[24,31]

The importance of support from senior leadership is essential for IPE and IPCP to not only survive but thrive in an organization. RWJF outlines some key practices that senior leadership must demonstrate in order to promote IPE in an organization.[24]

- Senior leaders need to create visible partnerships across disciplines so that employees see those in leadership modeling collaboration.
- Senior leaders need to identify champions of IPE and IPCP to serve as role models for the organization. These individuals should be highly visible so that others can see the behavior modeled in practice.
- It is also important to "embed goals into the strategic plan and tie them to the performance incentives of key leaders and influencers."[24(p23)] This ensures there are tangible measures of how senior leaders can support IPE and IPCP.
- Conflict is expected in any well-functioning organization. To support IPE and IPCP, it is recommended that any conflict should be debated in private, while a shared and equal voice should be used in public. This will demonstrate a united front and provide a role model for collaboration in the organization.

Though support from senior leadership is imperative, the organizational culture must also support IPE and IPCP in order for them to be accepted. Grymonpre and colleagues used the conceptual framework developed by D'Amour and Oandasan[32] to guide the implementation of IPE in their organization.[33] They identified the importance of creating an organizational structure to support IPE in order to integrate IPE and IPCP throughout the organization. In their academic setting, they appointed an IPE steering committee and an IPE coordinator. In a nonacademic setting, this could be a senior vice president who is accountable to the board of directors. This way not only do the senior leaders demonstrate a commitment to IPE and IPCP, but the organizational culture also incorporates this expectation. Grymonpre also recommends that organizations adopt inclusive terminology in an effort to "harmonize language, reduce confusion, and avoid misunderstanding between the academic and practice sectors."[33(p84)] It is also stressed that this common language should respect professional differences. This point supports the fact that IPE should be an integral part of the educational system so students understand and can use a common language once in practice.

Another component of acceptability is building interprofessional champions both in higher education and the health care system. In higher education, champions can be groomed and supported through faculty development.[31] Faculty development has been identified as a way to support both faculty and clinicians in modeling IPE and IPCP in daily practice.[33] Farnsworth and colleagues identified overall IPE success in an academic setting by surveying deans and faculty members. One of their conclusions stressed the importance of "positively incentivizing, training and formally recognizing faculty participation in IPE."[29(p156)] If faculty development is not supported, it is less likely that IPE will be integrated into the curriculum and thus modeled in clinical practice. Hall and Zierler evaluated their faculty development programs and stressed the importance of purposeful reflection to facilitate authentic debriefing instead of only task-oriented activities. Another interesting conclusion encouraged the use of vectors such as QI and patient safety as explicit topics, but ultimately teamwork is the implicit curriculum.[34]

In addition to support from senior leadership, faculty, and clinical staff; continuing educational opportunities; and human resources support, the relational nature of the interactions must be valued in order for IPE and IPCP to thrive. Even though it was a small qualitative study, Olson, Klupp, and Astell-Burt asked how interpersonal relationships influence IPE[35] by using Holland's theory of identities as practice[36] to analyze IPE in a university setting. One conclusion of the study stressed the importance of interprofessional friendships and relationships.[35] Since professional identities begin to form before formal education begins, having the opportunity to work with each other, work though problems, and develop respectful relationships may lead to more genuine relationships, which in turn break down barriers to collaboration. While these relationships occur while in the university setting, the respect and acceptance of other disciplines may transition to clinical practice.[24] To break down the barriers between disciplines and to promote shared decision making, the relational aspect of collaboration should be encouraged. In a clinical setting, this can be shared workspaces and case conferences where formal and informal interactions are encouraged.

Affordability (Economic)

There are many who suggest that health care should not be conducted as a business. However, there are financial implications that should be considered. The third component of the sustainable model is economics, or the **affordability** of IPE and IPCP. As with any endeavor, administrative support within the organization is essential. Financial support is usually discussed when prioritizing initiatives as well as some level of return on investment. Currently there is a lack of information available on the cost of IPE and IPCP as well as their value.[8] However, there is a need to conduct research in this area, especially since we know the detrimental effects of poor teamwork and communication.

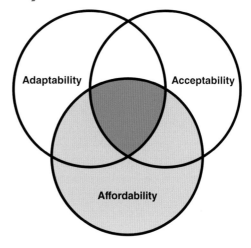

Lawlis and colleagues noted funding as an institutional enabler for IPE academic programs.[7] At this time, it is unknown whether an organizational structure with a centralized office or a combination of dedicated program-level faculty is more effective and efficient in the delivery of IPE. The same is true for health care delivery. Does the hospital or clinic office support a centralized office for IPCP, does each department have an individual team member focused on teamwork training, or are IPCP training and assessment integrated in a current employee education or quality assurance department? These are just some of the initial organizational questions related to costs that need to be discussed.

Carney and colleagues discuss 3 financing models for IPE within an academic university.[37] The first option provides a budget for a centralized IPE office. The centralized office coordinates, implements, and assesses IPE. The income derives from additional student tuition fees dedicated to IPE. These funds cover costs for faculty and staff salaries as well as normal departmental operations. Clinical environments do not typically bill patients for additional fees, not covered by insurance, to cover standard-of-care services. Therefore, this type of funding model would not be sustainable for most clinical settings.

The second option also charges additional fees to students, but the fee is lower because faculty members are not paid additional wages for IPE time.[37] Instead, faculty members are provided time within the current work week to support IPE efforts, and the idea of a centralized office still exists. Since this option also involves additional fees, it probably would not be viable for clinical environments.

The third option does not include additional fees or have a centralized office.[37] All departments have their own faculty focused on IPE and share costs associated with learning activities; there is no consistent entity that coordinates, implements, and assesses IPE. This third option could be an economic model for clinical environments because no additional fees are billed and each department has faculty dedicated to IPE efforts.

Having a discussion about financial support is essential because interprofessional training is required across multiple departments and programs. Funding is needed for faculty and staff time for the development, implementation, and assessment of IPE experiences, similar to a program-specific learning activity.[37] From an IPCP perspective, administrators will need to define costs associated with training and

COLLABORATIVE CORNER
Maximizing Implicit Coordination

To address the health needs of patients and communities, we must begin to maximize IPCP that does not require face-to-face communication among health care providers. Low-interdependence tasks, such as appropriate and timely consultations, are valuable forms of collaborative practice that can translate to lower costs for organizations. Take, for example, a patient who has been recently diagnosed with type II diabetes mellitus by an FNP. Based on the patient's needs, the FNP can refer the patient to a certified diabetic educator, an endocrinologist, a registered dietitian nutritionist, a support group, or a self-management education program for chronic disease. The act of referral requires the provider to understand the various roles of other clinicians, as well as the purpose and availability of community resources. Implicit coordination among the health team, which does not require face-to-face time, can influence affordability and improve the sustainability of IPCP.

practice. In the third funding option, the question of who will coordinate and assess the effects of training and implementation needs to be discussed. IPCP training may not be paid for prior to health care delivery, but it will be important to measure patient outcomes when care is rendered by interprofessional teams.

IPCP was recently recognized in the American Medical Association (AMA) book on Current Procedural Terminology (CPT). There are CPT billing codes for physician and qualified nonphysician providers engaging in IPCP. Reimbursable codes can assist with sustainability because there is payment for the time spent collaborating to improve patient outcomes. Codes 99446 through 99449, 99451, and 99452 are published in the *CPT 2019 Professional Edition*. These codes provide reimbursement for the treating provider and the consultant provider. It is important to educate health professionals on the availability of these billing codes to quantify IPCP time. With these data, services and health outcomes can be correlated with collaborative practice. The assessment of costs, health outcomes, patient satisfaction, and provider satisfaction related to IPCP is needed to sustain efforts.

Emerging Research and Opportunities for Interprofessional Growth

The majority of this book describes what is currently known in the IPE and IPCP arena. This concluding chapter reemphasizes the known but situates the content in an existing model focused on sustainability. As a health professional, it is important to understand what research has been conducted in both academic and clinical environments, because education will influence practice, and practice should influence the delivery of education.

It is equally important to stay abreast of emerging interprofessional research, which has the potential to support IPE and IPCP sustainability in the future. Three examples are the following:

1. *The meta-model of interprofessional development.*[40] Figure 8.3 describes the phases of interprofessional development as outlined by the authors of the model. This model has the potential to affect the development and timing of educational experiences.

2. *The interprofessional socialization framework.*[48-50] This framework provides a model for interprofessional socialization that helps students develop their dual identity. See the sidebar Theorized IPSF for more information.

3. *The Cs of team science.*[41] Figure 8.4 on page 181 highlights 7 aspects of teamwork that can be used by student and clinician teams to evaluate and improve their team effectiveness.

As champions in this area, be aware of new developments when attending conferences and reading scholarly work.

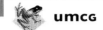
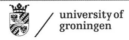
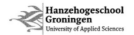
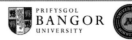
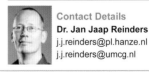
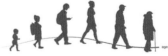

Figure 8.3 Meta-model for interprofessional development poster.
Courtesy of Dr. Jan Jaap Reinders.

THEORIZED IPSF: THREE STAGES OF INTERPROFESSIONAL SOCIALIZATION

Stage I: Breaking Down Barriers

- **The goal:** Assisting learners to modify their uniprofessional perspective by reducing or eliminating their out-group discrimination.
- **The process:** (1) Creating an open and trusting environment through the application of Pettigrew's[51] optimal contact conditions (equal status among the students and staff and cooperation towards setting and meeting common goals). (2) Breaking down barriers against interprofessional learning and collaboration through the incorporation of Pettigrew's[51] four interdependent cognitive processes (learning about out-groups, changing behavior, generating affective ties, and in-group reappraisal) using small group interprofessional interaction or discussion and critical reflection.
- **The outcome:** The development of an adjusted professional identity (with no out-group discrimination) in which perceived threats to professional identity are reduced, allowing and inspiring learners to begin learning with and from each other and to move towards developing interprofessional teamwork.

Stage II: Interprofessional Role Learning and Interprofessional Collaboration

- **The goal:** Cultivating the culture of IPC in which learners mutually value and respect the (complementary) roles and contributions of each profession to clients' care.
- **The process:** Engaging the learners in case study discussion while applying the interprofessional core competency domains including patient, client, family, and community-centered care; interprofessional communication, roles, and responsibilities; team and team functioning; interprofessional conflict resolution; values and ethics; and collaborative leadership.[52,53]
- **The outcome:** Mastering the IPC competencies enhances learners' shared decision-making and power-sharing capabilities resulting in the development of a sense of belonging and identity to the interprofessional team or community.[32]

Stage III: Dual Identity Development

- **The goal:** Transformation to dual identity that occurs when learners simultaneously identify themselves as part of their own profession and their interprofessional community.
- **The process:** The development of an interprofessional identity assists the learners to equally value, respect, and celebrate diverse contributions of each team member in client care as a unified team. Further in-depth

(continued)

Theorized IPSF: Three Stages of Interprofessional Socialization *(continued)*

critical reflection on their interprofessional partnership helps learners to embrace and develop a shared set of identities—professional and interprofessional or dual identity.

- **The outcome:** Learners embrace both adjusted professional identity (by eliminating their out-group discrimination) and a sense of interprofessionality (by extending their in-group status to include all), which leads to
  - maintaining their own professional solidarity,
  - reducing fear of identity loss, and
  - diminishing turf protection behaviors.

If sustained, the dual identity is theorized to increase learners' willingness to seek collaborative teamwork.

Reprinted by permission from H. Khalili, *Interprofessional Socialization and Dual Identity Development Amongst Cross-Disciplinary Students,* Dissertation (University of Western Ontario, London, Canada, 2013).

The health industry has much more to learn about IPE and IPCP, and there are many opportunities to advance your knowledge. Whether you are a student, faculty member, clinician, or administrator, if you are reading this book, we hope you join other champions in this area. We are all dedicated to discovering and employing evidence-based practices to improve the health of the communities we serve.

As a student or a recent student, you have had the unique opportunity to engage in IPE during formal academic training and have a foundation from which to grow interprofessionally. As a new clinician, you also have the ability to share new knowledge with your work teams. If you are a faculty member currently not engaged in IPE, consider developing internal relationships with faculty engaged in IPE and discover opportunities to partner with other academic departments. More experienced clinicians and administrators who do not have formal IPE training should contact their local college or university for opportunities to learn more. These professional relationships are mutually beneficial with bidirectional learning. Clinicians offer academic faculty a unique perspective of daily operations that facilitate or challenge IPCP. These daily occurrences are relevant learning activities for students and can enhance realism in case examples. Case examples are ideal opportunities for reflection and development in collaborative practice. So, continue to use the case studies and collaborative corners in each of the chapters to support your interprofessional development.

There are many stakeholders, both organizations and individuals, in the United States that support IPE and IPCP. Currently, IPE research is growing at a faster pace than IPCP research. Recognizing and responding to this gap within the interprofessional spectrum is critical as we continue to build support and sustainability for IPCP.

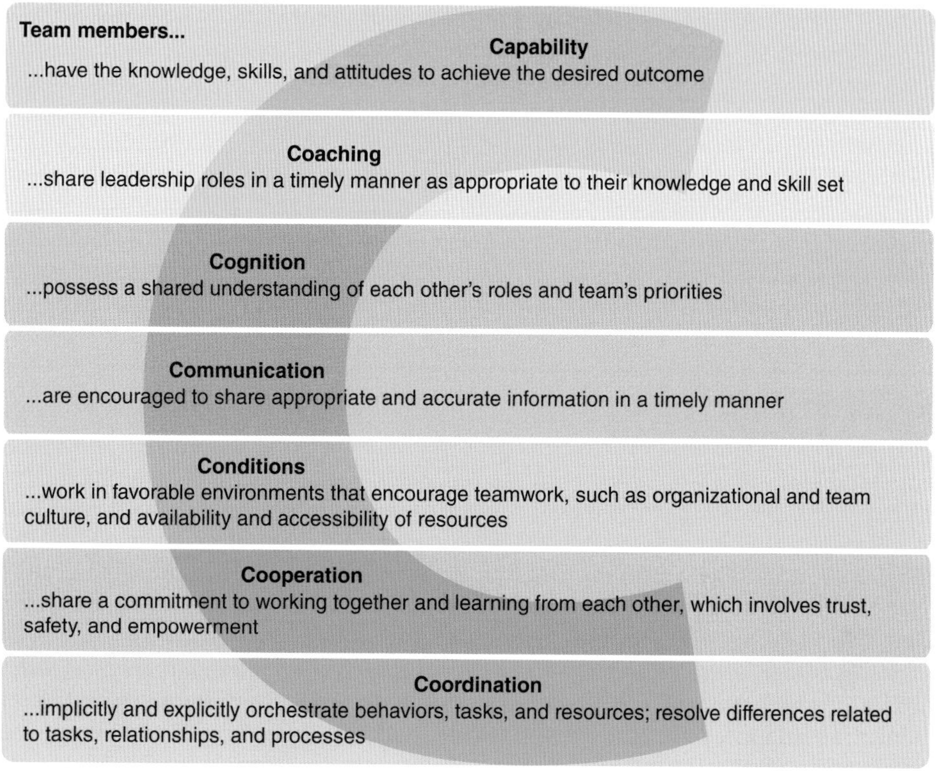

Team members...
Capability
...have the knowledge, skills, and attitudes to achieve the desired outcome

Coaching
...share leadership roles in a timely manner as appropriate to their knowledge and skill set

Cognition
...possess a shared understanding of each other's roles and team's priorities

Communication
...are encouraged to share appropriate and accurate information in a timely manner

Conditions
...work in favorable environments that encourage teamwork, such as organizational and team culture, and availability and accessibility of resources

Cooperation
...share a commitment to working together and learning from each other, which involves trust, safety, and empowerment

Coordination
...implicitly and explicitly orchestrate behaviors, tasks, and resources; resolve differences related to tasks, relationships, and processes

Figure 8.4   Team science Cs.

Summary

Interprofessional learning is a lifelong practice, beginning with acceptance into a health professional program, transitioning to advanced formal education opportunities, and continuing throughout one's career.[8] Developing appropriate and meaningful IPE opportunities throughout a career will be critical to maturing in IPCP. Academic, clinical, and continuing education organizations will need to collaborate on a lifelong continuum of education for health professionals, addressing the 3 pillars of sustainability.

Sustaining IPE and IPCP throughout the health industry will be foundational to improving health outcomes and providing affordable care. Administrators leading these initiatives should use the elements of a sustainable model (affordability, acceptability, and adaptability) when addressing needs and solutions. A comprehensive list of IPE enablers and barriers has been developed for academic organizations. Some IPE enablers, such as administrative financial support and acceptance from health professionals, will be similar for IPCP practice settings. However, differences between the settings do exist, such as curricula within academia and patient scheduling in clinical environments.

IPE and IPCP are highly dependent on each other. External organizations such as the Josiah Macy Jr. Foundation, RWJF, and HRSA have provided and will continue to provide support for team-based care (adaptability). However, administrators need to analyze organizational structure and work environments that socially (acceptability) and financially (affordability) support the efforts of a team, not a single profession or entity. Addressing the 3 elements of a sustainable model provides support for integration and "development that meets the needs of the present without compromising the ability of future generations to meet their own."[2 (p154)] IPE research is growing at a faster pace than IPCP research, and recognizing and responding to this gap is essential as we continue to build support and sustainability for IPCP.

CASE STUDY Debriefing

IPE is a lifelong learning process that requires support from educators, administrators, and staff. If IPCP supports improved health outcomes, then administrators should consider engaging QI offices for incorporation into existing structures. Most published research has been conducted by academic researchers focused on IPE. Therefore, it will be important for clinical environments to develop collaborative efforts with educational institutions to determine what to measure, how to measure, and how to progress learning in team-based care.

Valued-based care and reimbursement of patient outcomes are an influential driver of services. If IPCP support improves health outcomes, then integration of education and support systems for team-based care becomes imperative in the dynamic health care system.

Case Study Discussion Questions

1. If you are the consultant for Gold Health Care System, what recommendations would you suggest to initiate and sustain the IPCP initiative?
2. How will you identify the stakeholders in Gold Health Care System who will not only support the initiation of IPE and IPCP but help to sustain them within the organization?
3. How can IPE advancements in educational environments support collaborative practice within Gold Health Care System?
4. Are there any practice areas where IPE can be first implemented in order to increase buy-in from the providers, staff, and leaders?
5. What resources might Gold Health Care System use to support IPCP among health professionals?

Appendix

Additional Resources

African Interprofessional Education Network (AfrIPEN)

This Africa-based organization supports interprofessional education and collaborative practice.

Agency for Healthcare Research and Quality (AHRQ)

The agency's Team STEPPS program is an evidence-based set of teamwork tools aimed at optimizing patient outcomes by improving communication and teamwork skills among health care professionals.

American Interprofessional Health Collaborative (AIHC)

The American Interprofessional Health Collaborative provides learning opportunities and resources, including the Collaborating Across Borders Conference.

Australasian Interprofessional Practice & Education Network (AIPPEN)

This Australia and New Zealand-based organization supports integrated learning.

Canadian Interprofessional Health Collaborative

This Canada-based organization supports collaborative, patient-centered practice.

Centre for the Advancement of Interprofessional Education (CAIPE)

Based in the United Kingdom, this community of practice describes itself as a think tank supporting students, educators, practitioners, and researchers in interprofessional education.

Health, Interprofessional Practice & Education

This journal supports research in interprofessional education and collaborative practice.

Health Professions Accreditors Collaborative (HPAC)

This group of health care accreditors supports the development and implementation of IPE.

Indian Interprofessional Education Network (IndiPEN)

This India-based organization supports interprofessional education and collaborative practice.

Institute for Healthcare Improvement (IHI)

This institute authored the original Triple Aim framework for optimizing health system performance through three critical objectives.

Interprofessional Education Collaborative (IPEC)

Author of a set of core competencies, IPEC works in collaboration with academic institutions to promote workforce-ready graduates for interprofessional collaborative practices.

Interprofessional.Global: Global Confederation for Interprofessional Education & Collaborative Practice

This organization supports interaction among interprofessional education and collaborative practice networks across the globe.

Josiah Macy Jr. Foundation

This foundation focuses on improving the education of health professionals.

Journal of Interprofessional Care

This journal supports research in interprofessional education and collaborative practice.

Journal of Interprofessional Education and Practice

This journal supports research in interprofessional education and collaborative practice.

Journal of Research in Interprofessional Practice and Education

This journal supports research in interprofessional education and collaborative practice.

MedEdPORTAL

This is a peer-reviewed teaching and learning resource center.

National Academy of Medicine (NAM)

This organization focuses on improvements in health care quality and equity.

National Center for Interprofessional Practice and Education (NCIPE)

This is a unique public–private partnership that provides leadership, evidence, and resources to guide the nation on the use of interprofessional education and collaborative practice to enhance the experience of health care, improve population health, and reduce the overall cost of care.

National Collaborative for Improving the Clinical Learning Environment (NCICLE)

This collaborative brings together organizations for the improvement of the clinical education experience and patient outcomes in clinical environments.

Nordic Interprofessional Network (NIPNET)

This Scandanavia-based organization supports interprofessional education and collaborative practice.

Regional Network for Interprofessional Education in the Americas (REIP)

This Central America, South American, and Caribbean network supports interprofessional education and collaborative practice.

Robert Wood Johnson Foundation

This is a philanthropic organization that supports the health of all individuals.

World Health Organization

This is an international organization that supports health within the United Nations system.

Glossary

A3—A 1-page (A3 size) tool that guides the user through a problem-solving process using the scientific method.

acceptability—The pillar of sustainability that addresses how to promote IPCP and IPE buy-in from clinicians, administrators, staff, and patients.

adaptability—The pillar of sustainability that addresses both the internal and external organizational elements necessary to IPE and IPCP.

affective skills—Skills related to understanding and communicating feelings and emotions related to self and others; in health care professions, includes the expression of sympathy or empathy in patient care.

affordability—The pillar of sustainability that addresses how financial support is necessary to sustain IPE and IPCP in an organization.

asynchronous activity—A learning activity that happens at a time that is convenient for the learner, in a singular fashion.

blended IPE—Providing material online that is studied before a face-to-face meeting where the actual IPE engagement will occur.

brief—A short, intentional gathering of multiple health care professionals prior to an experience to establish a plan and next steps.

briefing—A structure for communication that can be implemented in a variety of IPE activities.

bypassing—When members of a team assume that everyone on the team understands what is being said.

cognitive skills—Skills the brain uses to read, think, problem solve, and collaborate on teams; in health care professions, includes the knowledge of professional practice.

collaborative practice-ready health workforce—Health care professionals who work together to provide comprehensive services in various settings.

cross-boundary teaming—Individuals with differences in expertise and organization form a temporary group tasked with quickly developing into an effective and efficient team to address a novel project.

debriefing—A structure for reflection that can be implemented in a variety of IPE activities.

direct health care provider—A health care provider who directly interacts with the patient, such as a bedside nurse.

dual identity—Identity that develops through exposure to learning experiences that promote both uniprofessional and interprofessional socialization and competency.

facial expression and eye behavior—A form of nonverbal language that tells the emotional state of both listeners and speakers.

facilitation—The process of helping groups or individuals to learn, find solutions, or reach consensus without imposing or dictating an outcome.

faculty champions—Educators who lead by example to create change around a specific initiative.

gray literature—Any literature that is neither peer reviewed nor published in peer-reviewed journals and is available through indexed databases for review; examples include white papers, bulletins, and technical reports.

health and education systems—Organizations, people, and actions whose primary intent is to promote, restore, or maintain health and facilitate learning, respectively.

health worker—Person whose primary intent is to enhance health, or one who promotes and preserves health, diagnoses and treats disease, performs health management, and supports workers, as well as others who contribute to the overall health or wellness of a person or group of people. For this book, these are further defined as the professionals who provide direct health care (whether primary or rehabilitative) and may include physicians, nurses, OTs, speech therapists, PTs, athletic trainers, nutritionists, social workers, and physician assistants (PAs).

indirect health care provider—A health care employee who provides services that support direct care providers, such as a nurse working in health informatics.

interprofessional collaborative practice (IPCP)—When health care providers of varying professions work together with patients, families, caregivers, and communities to deliver quality care.

interprofessional education (IPE)—When two or more professions learn about, from, and with each other to enable IPCP and improve health outcomes. The goal of IPE is a collaborative practice-ready health workforce.

interprofessional professionalism—Demonstrating core values as a health care professional working with others to achieve health and wellness in individuals and communities.

interprofessional team-based care—Care delivered by health care work groups that have a collective identity and shared responsibility for patients.

interprofessional teamwork—Cooperation, coordination, and collaboration between professions in delivering patient-centered care.

kinesthetics—A form of nonverbal language composed of body language and gestures to communicate messages.

knowledge diversity—The varying professional experiences, educational experiences, and perspectives in a group with members of different professions and professional roles.

leading indicators—Process measures typically gathered through manual data collection. An example might be an observation. Process measures are commonly used as leading indicators.

multiprofessional education (MPE)—The process by which a group of students (or workers) in health-related fields and with different educational backgrounds learn together during certain periods of their education. MPE is generally thought of as a precursor to IPE and IPCP.

outcome measures—Measures that quantify the output of a process; typically easy to collect due to often being found in electronic systems but can be hard to improve or influence.

paralinguistics—A form of nonverbal language including the speaker's pitch, volume, and junctures.

process measures—Measures that quantify specific steps in a process; typically difficult to collect due to the manual nature of data collection (i.e., observation) but useful in understanding cause-and-effect relationships in a process.

proxemics—A form of nonverbal language that is concerned with the use of space for communication.

psychological safety—Perceived consequences of taking interpersonal risks.

Robert's Rules of Order—A guide outlining common rules (parliamentary procedure) for leading a meeting or team through deliberation, debate, and respectful communication.

scoping review—A type of review that maps the existing literature in a topic area to examine the extent, range, and nature of research activity.

sister meetings—Scheduling separate meetings to address a topic for group members who work complementary schedules (e.g., a meeting for day-shift members during the day and then the same meeting with shared content for the night-shift members).

Six Sigma—Disciplined approach to solving problems that focuses on eliminating defects through minimizing variation.

soft skills—Personal traits or attributes that enable people to effectively interact with others.

sustainability—The ability to develop in a way that meets present needs without compromising the ability to meet future ones.

synchronous activity—A learning activity that happens at a specific time in a group with course peers and instructors.

team—A group of people working together to complete a job, task, or project with a mutual goal.

teaming—An active process of working together.

Team Oriented Problem Solving (TOPS)—Multifaceted problem-solving strategy that requires at minimum 4 participants from 4 organizational areas who methodically apply 8 disciplines.

TeamSTEPPS—Tools for teamwork to improve communication and teamwork skills among health care professionals, thus optimizing patient outcomes.

True North goal—A central, meaningful, and impactful goal for the organization that is critical for developing effective health care teams.

References

Chapter 1

1. *Interprofessional Collaborative Practice in Healthcare, Getting Prepared, Preparing to Succeed.* www.elsevier.com/clinical-solutions/insights/resources/insights-articles/clinical-practice/interprofessional-collaborative-practice-in-healthcare. Accessed April 22, 2018.

2. Greiner AC, Knebel E, eds. *Health Professions Education: A Bridge to Quality.* Washington, DC: National Academies Press; 2003.

3. Joint Commission on Accreditation of Healthcare Organizations. National Patient Safety Goals. www.jointcommission.org/PatientSafety/NationalPatientSafetyGoals. Accessed April 22, 2018.

4. Reeves S, Perrier L, Goldman J, Freeth D, Zwarenstein M. Interprofessional education: effects on professional practice and health care outcomes (update). *Cochrane Database Syst Rev.* 2013;3:CD002213.

5. World Health Organization (WHO). Framework for Action on Interprofessional Education and Collaborative Practice. Geneva, Switzerland: WHO; 2010.

6. Frenk J, Chen L, Bhutta ZA, et al. Health professions for a new century: transforming education to strengthen health systems in an interdependent world. *Lancet.* 2010;376:1923-1958.

7. Homeyer S, Hoffmann W, Hingst P, Opperman R, Dreier-Wolfgramm A. Effects of IPE for medical and nursing students: enablers, barriers and expectations for optimizing future IP collaboration—a qualitative study. *BMC Nurs.* 2018;17:13.

8. Hoffman S, Rosenfield D, Gilbert JH, Oandasan IF. Student leadership in interprofessional education: benefits, challenges and implications for educators, researchers and policymakers. *Med Educ.* 2008;42(7):654-661.

9. Mitchell P, Belza B, Schaad D, et al. Working across the boundaries of health professions disciplines in education, research, and service: The University of Washington experience. *Academic Med.* 2006;81(10):891-896.

10. Bennet PN, Gum L, Lindeman I, Lawn S, McAllister S, Richards J, Kelton M, Ward H. Faculty perceptions of interprofessional education. *Nurse Educ Today.* 2010;31:571-576.

11. Chambers R, Tullys T, Mayer K, Wigand D. Regional collaborative practice in psychiatric rehabilitation and recovery: a best practice model. *J Social Work in Disability and Rehab.* 2008;7(3-4):187-231.

12. Brandt BF. Interprofessional education and collaborative practice: welcome to the "new" forty-year old field. https://nexusipe.org/informing/resource-center/interprofessional-education-and-collaborative-practice-welcome-new-forty. Accessed June 26, 2018.

13. Braithwaite J, Clay-Williams R, Vecellio E, Marks D, Hooper T, Westbrook M, Westbrook J, Blakely B, Ludlow K. The basis of clinical tribalism, hierarchy and stereotyping: a laboratory-controlled teamwork experiment. *BMJ Open.* 2016;6:e012467.

14. Clark K. Interprofessional education: making our way out of the silos. *Resp Care.* 2018;63:639.

15. Cox M, Blouin AS, Cuff P, Paniagua M, Philips S, Vlasses P. The role of accreditation in achieving the quadruple aim. NAM Perspectives. National Academy of Medicine.

https://nam.edu/the-role-of-accreditation-in-achieving-the-quadruple-aim. Accessed June 26, 2018.

16. Makary M. Operating room teamwork among physicians and nurses: teamwork in the eye of the beholder. *J Am Coll Surg*. 2006;202:746-752.

17. Brandt, BF. Interprofessional education and collaborative practice: welcome to the "new" forty-year old field. https://nexusipe.org/informing/resource-center/interprofessional-education-and-collaborative-practice-welcome-new-forty. Accessed June 26, 2018.

18. Baldwin D. Some historical notes on interdisciplinary and interprofessional education and practice in health care in the U.S.A. *J Interprof Care*. 1996;10:187-201.

19. National Academies of Sciences, Engineering, and Medicine (NASEM). 2017. Exploring the role of accreditation in enhancing quality and innovation in health professions education: proceedings of a workshop. Washington, DC: National Academies Press. doi:10.17226/23636

20. Institute of Medicine (IOM). *Health Professions Education: A Bridge to Quality*. Washington, DC: National Academies Press; 2003. doi:10.17226/10681

21. Robert Wood Johnson Foundation (RWJF). Lessons from the field: promising interprofessional collaboration practices. www.rwjf.org/en/library/research/2015/03/lessons-from-the-field.html. Accessed January 10, 2019.

22. American Interprofessional Health Collaborative (AIHC). AIHC website. What is AIHC? https://aihc-us.org/what-is-aihc. Accessed June 2, 2019.

23. Interprofessional Education Collaborative (IPEC). About IPEC. www.ipecollaborative.org/about-ipec.html. Accessed June 2, 2019.

24. Health Professions Accreditors Collaborative (HPAC). *Guidance on Developing Quality Interprofessional Education for the Health Professions*. https://nexusipe-summit.s3.us-west-2.amazonaws.com/2019/2019-01/HPAC-National-Center-GuidanceWeb-1.pdf. Accessed June 26, 2019.

25. World Health Organization (WHO). Learning together to work together for health. Geneva, Switzerland: WHO; 1988.

26. National Collaborative for Improving the Clinical Learning Environment (NCICLE). About NCICLE. https://nexusipe.org/informing/about-national-center Accessed September 16, 2019.

Chapter 2

1. World Health Organization (WHO). Framework for Action on Interprofessional Education and Collaborative Practice. Geneva, Switzerland: WHO; 2010.

2. Hall P. Interprofessional teamwork: professional cultures as barriers. *J Interprof Care*. 2005;19(suppl):188-196.

3. Oandasan I, Reeves S. Key elements for interprofessional education. Part 1: the learner, the educator and the learning context. *J Interprof Care*. 2005;19(suppl 1):21-38.

4. Health Professions Accreditors Collaborative (HPAC). (2019). *Guidance on Developing Quality Interprofessional Education for the Health Professions*. Chicago, IL: HPAC.

5. Barr, H. Toward a theoretical framework for interprofessional education. *J Interprof Care*. 2013;27(1):4-9.

6. Yamani N, Asgarimoqadam M, Haghani F, Alavijeh AQ. The effect of interprofessional education on interprofessional performance and diabetes care knowledge of health care teams at the level one of health service providing. *Adv Biomed Res*. 2014;3:153.

7. Feng J, Ying YT, Chang HY, Erdley WS, Lin CH, Chang YJ. Systematic review of effectiveness of situated e-learning on medical and nursing education. *Worldviews Evid Based Nurs.* 2013;10(3):174-183.

8. Salas E, Lazzara E, Benishek L, King H. On being a team player: Evidence-based heuristic for teamwork in interprofessional education. *Med Sci Educ.* 2013;23(3S):524-531.

9. Orchard, C, Rykhoff, M. Collaborative leadership within interprofessional practice. In: Forman D, Jones M, Thistlethwaite J, eds. *Leadership and Collaboration.* London, UK: Palgrave Macmillan; 2015:71-94.

10. Lamb G, Shraiky J. Designing for competence: spaces that enhance collaboration readiness in healthcare. *J Interprof Care.* 2013;27(suppl 2):14-23.

11. Masten Y, Acton C, Ashcraft A, Esperat C. Interprofessional education development: a road map for getting there. *Open J Nurs.* 2013;3(3):7.

12. Interprofessional Education Collaborative (IPEC). *Core Competencies for Interprofessional Collaborative Practice: 2016 Update.* Washington, DC: IPEC; 2016.

13. Eichbaum Q. Collaboration and teamwork in the health professions: rethinking the role of conflict. *Acad Med.* 2018;93(4):574-580.

14. Gilbert JH. The global emergence of IPE and collaborative care. *J Interprof Care.* 2010;24(5):473-474.

15. Steinert Y. Learning together to teach together: interprofessional education and faculty development. *J Interprof Care.* 2005;19(suppl 1):60-75.

16. Clark P. What would a theory of interprofessional education look like? Some suggestions for developing a theoretical framework for teamwork training. *J Interprof Care.* 2006;20(6):577-589.

17. Abu-Rish E, Kim S, Choe L, et al. Current trends in interprofessional education of health sciences students: a literature review. *J Interprof Care.* 2012;26(6):444-451.

18. West C, Graham L, Palmer RT, et al. Implementation of interprofessional education (IPE) in 16 U.S. medical schools: common practices, barriers and facilitators. *J Interprof Educ Pract.* 2016;4:41-49.

19. Zorek J, Raehl C. Interprofessional education accreditation standards in the USA: a comparative analysis. *J Interprof Care.* 2013;27(2):123-130.

20. Bodenheimer T, Sinsky C. From triple to quadruple aim: care of the patient requires care of the provider. *Ann Fam Med.* 2014;12(6):573-576.

21. Sargeant J, Hill T, Breau L. Development and testing of a scale to assess interprofessional education (IPE) facilitation skills. *J Contin Educ Health Prof.* 2010;30(2):126-131.

22. Rosen MA, DiazGranados D, Dietz AS, et al. Teamwork in healthcare: key discoveries enabling safer, high-quality care. *Am Psychol.* 2018;73(4):433-450.

23. Fiscella K, McDaniel SH. The complexity, diversity, and science of primary care teams. *Am Psychol.* 2018;73(4):451-467.

24. Dewey J. *How We Think: A Restatement of the Relation of Reflective Thinking to the Educational Process.* Vol 35. Lexington, MA: Heath; 1933.

25. Clapper TC, Ching K, Lee JG, et al. A TeamSTEPPS implementation plan for recently assigned interns and nurses. *J Interprof Care.* January 2019:1-5.

26. Agency for Healthcare Research and Quality (AHRQ). Team STEPPS. www.ahrq.gov/teamstepps/index.html. 2019.

27. Buring SM, Bhushan A, Broeseker A, et al. Interprofessional education: definitions, student competencies, and guidelines for implementation. *Am J Pharm Educ.* 2009;73(4):59.

28. Patel Gunaldo T, Brisolara KF, Davis AH, Moore R. Aligning interprofessional education collaborative sub-competencies to a progression of learning. *J Interprof Care.* 2017;31(3):394-396.

29. Thistlethwaite J, Moran M, World Health Organization Study Group on Interprofessional Education and Collaborative Practice. Learning outcomes for interprofessional education (IPE): literature review and synthesis. *J Interprof Care.* 2010;24(5):503-513.

30. Institute of Medicine (IOM). *Measuring the Impact of Interprofessional Education on Collaborative Practice and Patient Outcomes.* Washington DC: National Academies Press; 2015.

31. Kvan T. Evaluating learning environments for interprofessional care. *J Interprof Care.* 2013;27(suppl 2):31-36.

32. West C, Landry K, Graham A, et al. Conceptualizing interprofessional teams as multi-team systems—implications for assessment and training *Teach Learn Med.* 2015;27(4):366-369.

33. Gergerich E, Boland D, Scott MA. Hierarchies in interprofessional training. *J Interprof Care.* November 2018:1-8.

34. Pecukonis E, Doyle O, Acquavita S, Aparicio E, Gibbons M, Vanidestine T. Interprofessional leadership training in MCH social work. *Soc Work Health Care.* 2013;52(7):625-641.

35. Edmondson A. Psychological safety and learning behavior in work teams. *Adm Sci Q.* 1999;44(2):350-383.

36. O'Leary DF. Exploring the importance of team psychological safety in the development of two interprofessional teams. *J Interprof Care.* 2016;30(1):29-34.

37. Hean S, Craddock D, Hammick M. Theoretical insights into interprofessional education. *Med Teach.* 2012;34(2):158-160.

38. Hean S, Green C, Anderson E, et al. The contribution of theory to the design, delivery, and evaluation of interprofessional curricula: BEME Guide No. 49. *Med Teach.* 2018;40(6):542-558.

39. Fewster-Thuente L, Batteson T. Teaching collaboration competencies to healthcare provider students through simulation. *J Allied Health.* 2016;45(2):147-151.

40. Hammick M, Freeth D, Koppel I, Reeves S, Barr H. A best evidence systematic review of interprofessional education: BEME Guide No. 9. *Med Teach.* 2007;29(8):735-751.

41. Eliot KA, Breitbach AP, Toomey E, Hinyard L. The effectiveness of an introductory interprofessional course in building readiness for collaboration in the health professions. *Health Interprof Pract.* 2018;3(3).

42. Lairamore C, Morris D, Schichtl R, et al. Impact of team composition on student perceptions of interprofessional teamwork: a 6-year cohort study. *J Interprof Care.* 2018;32(2):143-150.

43. Dahlgren MA, Gustavsson M, Fejes A. Special issue: professional practice, education and learning: a sociomaterial perspective. *Stud Contin Educ.* 2018;40(3):239-241.

44. Carlisle C, Cooper H, Watkins C. "Do none of you talk to each other?": The challenges facing the implementation of interprofessional education. *Med Teach.* 2004;26(6):545-552.

45. Reeves S. *Developing and Delivering Practice-Based Interprofessional Education: Successes and Challenges* [dissertation]. London, UK: Institute of Health Sciences, City University; 2005.

46. Eliot K, Breitbach A, Wilson M, Chushak M. Institutional readiness for interprofessional education among nutrition and dietetics and athletic training education programs. *J Allied Health.* 2017;46(2):94-103.

47. McCutcheon LRM, Alzghari SK, Lee YR, Long WG, Marquez R. Interprofessional education and distance education: a review and appraisal of the current literature. *Curr Pharm Teach Learn.* 2017;9(4):729-736.

48. Reeves S, Pelone F, Harrison R, Goldman J, Zwarenstein M. Interprofessional collaboration to improve professional practice and healthcare outcomes. *Cochrane Database Syst Rev.* 2017;6:CD000072.

49. Thistlethwaite J. Interprofessional education: a review of context, learning and the research agenda. *Med Educ.* 2012;46(1):58-70.

50. Farnan JM, Gaffney S, Poston JT, et al. Patient safety room of horrors: a novel method to assess medical students and entering residents' ability to identify hazards of hospitalisation. *BMJ Qual Saf.* 2016;25(3):153-158.

51. Breitbach AP, Richardson R, National Athletic Trainers' Association Executive Committee for Education, Interprofessional Education and Practice in Athletic Training Work Group. Interprofessional education and practice in athletic training. *Athl Train Educ J.* April-June 2015;10(2):170-182

52. Reeves S, Fletcher S, Barr H, et al. A BEME systematic review of the effects of interprofessional education: BEME Guide No. 39. *Med Teach.* 2016;38(7):656-668.

53. Eliot KA, Breitbach AP, Hinyard L, Toomey E. The effectiveness of an introductory interprofessional course in building readiness for collaboration in the health professions. *Health Interprof Pract.* 2018;3(3).

54. Bultas MW, Ruebling I, Breitbach A, Carlson J. Views of the United States healthcare system: findings from documentary analysis of an interprofessional education course. *J Interprof Care.* 2016;30(6):762-768.

55. Hallin K, Kiessling A, Waldner A, Henriksson P. Active interprofessional education in a patient based setting increases perceived collaborative and professional competence. *Med Teach.* 2009;31(2):151-157.

56. Fowler TO, Wise HH, Mauldin MP, et al. Alignment of an interprofessional student learning experience with a hospital quality improvement initiative. *J Interprof Care.* April 2018:1-10.

57. Hendricks-Ferguson VL, Ruebling I, Sargeant DM, et al. Undergraduate students' perspectives of healthcare professionals' use of shared decision-making skills. *J Interprof Care.* March 2018:1-9.

58. Aronoff N, Stellrecht E, Lyons AG, et al. Teaching evidence-based practice principles to prepare health professions students for an interprofessional learning experience. *J Med Libr Assoc.* 2017;105(4):376-384.

59. Hall P, Brajtman S, Weaver L, Grassau PA, Varpio L. Learning collaborative teamwork: an argument for incorporating the humanities. *J Interprof Care.* 2014;28(6):519-525.

60. Pole D, Breitbach AP, Howell TG. Using a real-life case scenario to integrate additional health professions students into an existing interprofessional team seminar. *J Interprof Care.* 2016;30(2):242-244.

61. Fung L, Boet S, Bould MD, et al. Impact of crisis resource management simulation-based training for interprofessional and interdisciplinary teams: a systematic review. *J Interprof Care.* 2015;29(5):433-444.

62. Shrader S, Zaudke J, Jernigan S. An interprofessional objective structured teaching experience (iOSTE): an interprofessional preceptor professional development activity. *J Interprof Care*. 2018;32(1):98-100.

63. Kraft S, Wise HH, Jacques PF, Burik JK. Discharge planning simulation: training the interprofessional team for the future workplace. *J Allied Health*. 2013;42(3):175-181.

64. Housley CL, Neill KK, White LS, Tedder AT, Castleberry AN. An evaluation of an interprofessional practice-based learning environment using student reflections. *J Interprof Care*. 2018;32(1):108-110.

65. Uhlig PN, Doll J, Brandon K, et al. Interprofessional practice and education in clinical learning environments: frontlines perspective. *Acad Med*. 2018;93(10):1441-1444.

66. Harada ND, Traylor L, Rugen KW, et al. Interprofessional transformation of clinical education: the first six years of the Veterans Affairs Centers of Excellence in Primary Care Education. *J Interprof Care*. 2018:1-9.

67. Boet S, Bould MD, Layat Burn C, Reeves S. Twelve tips for a successful interprofessional team-based high-fidelity simulation education session. *Med Teach*. 2014;36(10):853-857.

68. Sweeney Haney T, Kott K, Rutledge CM, Britton B, Fowler CN, Poston RD. How to prepare interprofessional teams in two weeks: an innovative education program nested in telehealth. *Int J Nurs Educ Scholarsh*. January 2018;15(1).

69. Osborne ML, Tilden VP, Eckstrom E. Training health professions preceptors in rural practices: a challenge for interprofessional practice and education. *J Interprof Care*. April 2018:1-3.

70. Shrader S, Zaudke J. Top ten best practices for interprofessional precepting. *J Interprof Educ Pract*. 2018;10:56-60.

71. Milot E, Museux AC, Careau E. Facilitator training program: the Universite Laval interprofessional initiative. *Soc Work Health Care*. 2017;56(3):202-214.

72. Welsch LA, Hoch J, Poston RD, Parodi VA, Akpinar-Elci M. Interprofessional education involving didactic TeamSTEPPS and interactive healthcare simulation: a systematic review. *J Interprof Care*. 2018:1-9.

73. Brown DK, Wong AH, Ahmed RA. Evaluation of simulation debriefing methods with interprofessional learning. *J Interprof Care*. July 2018:1-3.

74. Salas E. Saving lives: The science of teamwork and what matters in practice. Presentation at Louisiana State University Health-New Orleans.

Chapter 3

1. Watkins K. Faculty development to support interprofessional education in healthcare professions: a realist approach. *J Interp Care*. 2016;30(6):695-701.

2. Rutherford-Hemming T, Lioce L. State of interprofessional education in nursing: a systematic review. *Nurse Educ*. 2018;43(1):9-13.

3. Masoomi R. What is the best evidence medical education. *Research Develop Med Educ*. 2012;1:3-5

4. Thistlethwaite JE. Interprofessional education: implications and development for medical education. *Educ Med*. 2015;16:68-73.

5. Steinert Y. Learning together to teach together: interprofessional education and faculty development. *J Inter Care*. 2005;19(suppl):60-75.

6. Pemberton J, Rambaran M, Cameron BH. Evaluating the long-term impact of the Trauma Team Training course in Guyana: an explanatory mixed-methods approach. *Am J Surg*. 2013;205:119-124.

7. Hall P, Brajtman S, Weaver L, Grassau PA, Varpio L. Learning collaborative teamwork: an argument for incorporating the humanities. *J Interprof Care*. 2014;28:519-525.

8. Morgan P, Tregunno D, Brydges R, Pittini R, Tarshis J, Kurrek M, DeSousa S, Ryzynski A. Using a situational awareness global assessment technique for interprofessional obstetrical team training with high fidelity simulation. *J Interprof Care*. 2015;29:13-19.

9. Rozmus, CL, Carlin, N, Polczynski, A, Spike, J, Buday, R. The Brewsters: A new resource for interprofessional ethics education. *Nurs Ethics*. 2015;22:815-826.

10. World Health Organization (WHO). Framework for Action on Interprofessional Education and Collaborative Practice. Geneva, Switzerland: WHO; 2010.

11. Kirkpatrick DL, Kirkpatrick JD. *Evaluating Training Programs: The Four Levels*. 3rd ed. San Francisco, CA: Berrett-Koehler; 2006.

12. Ralyea, CM. *For Labor and Delivery Staff, How Does the Implementation of TeamSTEPPS Compared to Current Practice Impact Quality Indicators Over a Six-Month Period?* [dissertation]. Minneapolis: Capella University; 2013.

13. Rotz, ME, Dueñas, GG, Zanoni, A, Grover, AB. Designing and evaluating an interprofessional experiential course involving medical and pharmacy students. *Am J Pharm Educ*. 2016;80:85.

14. Interprofessional Education Collaborative Expert Panel (IPECEP). Core competencies for interprofessional collaborative practice: report of an expert panel. Washington, DC: IPEC; 2011.

15. Institute of Medicine (IOM). *Health Professions Education: A Bridge to Quality*. Washington, DC: National Academies Press; 2003. doi:10.17226/10681

16. Buring S, Bhushan A, Brazeau G, Conway S, Hansen L, Westberg S. Keys to successful implementation of interprofessional education: learning location, faculty development and curricular themes. *Am J Pharm Educ*. 2009;73(4):Article 60.

17. Harden RM. The integration ladder: a tool for curriculum planning and evaluation. *Med Educ*. 2000;34(7):551-557.

18. Anderson ES, Cox D, Thorpe LN. Preparation of educators involved in interprofessional education. *J Interprof Care*. 2009;23(1):81-94.

19. Poirier T, Wilhelm M. An interprofessional faculty seminar focused on interprofessional education. *Am J Pharm Educ*. 2014;78(4):Article 80.

20. Anderson ES, Thorpe LN, Hammick M. Interprofessional staff development: changing attitudes and winning hearts and minds. *J Interprof Care*. 2011;25(1):11-17.

21. Zook SS, Hulton LJ, Dudding CC, Stewart AL, Graham AC. Scaffolding interprofessional education: unfolding case studies, virtual world simulations and patient-centered care. *Nurse Educ*. 2018;43(2):87-91.

22. Olenick M, Allen LR. Faculty intent to engage in interprofessional education. *J Multidiscip Healthc*. 2013;19(6):149-161.

23. Al-Qahtani M, Guraya S. Measuring the attitudes of healthcare faculty members towards interprofessional education in KSA. *J Taibah Univ Med Sci*. 2016;11(6):586-593.

24. Giordano C, Elena U, Kevin JL. Attitudes of faculty and students in medicine and the health professions towards interprofessional education. *J Allied Health*. 2012;41(1):21-15.

25. Bassendowski S, Layne J, Lee L, Hupaelo T. Supporting clinical preceptors with interprofessional orientation sessions. *J Applied Health*. 2010;39(1):e23-e28.

26. Petersen CL, Callahan MF, McCarthy DO, Hughes RG, White-Traut R, Bansal NK. An online educational program improves pediatric oncology nurses' knowledge, attitudes, and spiritual care competence. *J Pediatr Oncol Nurs.* 2017;34(2):130-139.

27. Curran V, Casimiro L, Banfield V, et al. Interprofessional Collaborator Assessment Rubric. Academic Health Council. www.med.mun.ca/getdoc/b78eb859-6c13-4f2f-9712-f50f1c67c863/ICAR.aspx. Accessed October 23, 2015.

28. Bilodeau A, Dumont S, Hagan L, et al. Interprofessional education at Laval University: building an integrated curriculum for patient-centered practice. *J Interprof Care.* 2010;24(5):524-535.

29. Parsell G, Bligh, J. The development of a questionnaire to assess the readiness of health care students for interprofessional learning (RIPLS). *Med Educ.* 1999;33(2):95-100.

30. Reid R, Bruce D, Allstaff K, McLernon D. Validating the Readiness for Interprofessional Learning Scale (RIPLS) in the postgraduate context: are health care professionals ready for IPL? *Med Educ.* 2006;40(5):415-422.

31. World Health Organization (WHO). Framework for Action on Interprofessional Education and Collaborative Practice. Geneva, Switzerland: WHO; 2013.

32. National Academies of Sciences, Engineering, and Medicine (NASEM). *Exploring the Role of Accreditation in Enhancing Quality and Innovation in Health Professions Education: Proceedings of a Workshop.* Washington, DC: National Academies Press; 2017. doi:10.17226/23636

33. Commission on Accreditation of Athletic Training Education (CAATE). *Standards for the Accreditation of Post-Professional Athletic Training Degree Programs.* Austin, TX: CAATE; 2013.

34. Accreditation Council for Education in Nutrition and Dietetics (ACEND). ACEND 2017 Accreditation Standards. 2017. www.eatrightpro.org/-/media/eatrightpro-files/acend/about-program-accreditation/accreditation-standards/2017-standardsforcpprograms.pdf?la=en&hash=3D7E7EA5436607BD5A16917355ED50D32ED9CF92. Accessed March 25, 2019.

35. American Association of Colleges of Nursing (AACN). *The Essentials of Doctoral Education for Advanced Nursing Practice.* Washington, DC: AACN; 2006.

36. Accreditation Council for Occupational Therapy Education (ACOTE). 2011 Accreditation Council for Occupational Therapy Education (ACOTE) standards. *Am J Occup Ther.* November/December 2012;66:S6-S74. doi:10.5014/ajot.2012.66S6

37. Accreditation Council for Pharmacy Education (ACPE). *Accreditation Standards and Key Elements for the Professional Program in Pharmacy Leading to the Doctor of Pharmacy Degree.* 2016. www.acpe-accredit.org/pdf/Standards2016FINAL.pdf. Accessed March 25, 2019.

38. Commission on Accreditation in Physical Therapy Education (CAPTE). *Standards and Required Elements for Accreditation of Physical Therapy Education Programs.* www.capteonline.org/AccreditationHandbook. Accessed March 25, 2019.

39. Accreditation Review Commission on Education for the Physician Assistant, Inc. (ARC-PA). *Accreditation Standards for the Physician Assistant Profession.* 2018. www.arc-pa.org/wp-content/uploads/2018/06/Standards-4th-Ed-March-2018.pdf. Accessed March 25, 2019.

40. Council for Clinical Certification in Audiology and Speech-Language Pathology of the American Speech-Language-Hearing Association. 2014 Standards for the Certificate of Clinical Competence in Speech-Language Pathology. www.asha.org/Certification/2014-Speech-Language-Pathology-Certification-Standards. Accessed March 25, 2019.

41. Cox M, Naylor M. *Transforming Patient Care: Aligning Interprofessional Education with Clinical Practice Redesign*. Josiah Macy Jr. Foundation postconference report. New York, NY: Josiah Macy Jr. Foundation; 2013.

42. McKimm J, Swanwick T. Web-based faculty development: e-learning for clinical teachers in the London Deanery. *Clin Teach*. 2010;7(1):58-62.

43. Sargeant J, Hill T, Breau L. Development and testing of a scale to assess interprofessional education (IPE) facilitation skills. *J Cont Educ Health Prof*. 2010;30(2):126-131.

44. Hall L, Zierler B. Interprofessional education and practice guide no. 1: developing faculty to effectively facilitate interprofessional education. *J Inter Care*. 2015;29:3-7.

45. Kwan D, Barker KK, Austin Z, et al. Effectiveness of a faculty development program on interprofessional education: a randomized controlled trial. *J Interprof Care*. 2006;20(3):314-316.

46. Shrader S, Mauldin M, Hammad S, Mitcham M, Blue A. Developing a comprehensive faculty development program to promote interprofessional education, practice and research at a free-standing academic health science center. *J Inter Care*. 2015;29:165-167.

47. Medves J, Van Dijk J, Edgelow M, Saxe-Braithwaite M, working group of the IPECWG. *Pre-Registration Strategies to Guide the Teaching and Assessment of Interprofessional Competencies in IPE Settings. Report #3 of the Interprofessional Education Curricula Models for Health Care Providers in Ontario Working Group to the Interprofessional Care Strategic Implementation Committee*. Kingston, Ontario: Queen's University; 2009.

48. Toner JA, Ferguson KD, Sokal RD. Continuing interprofessional education in geriatrics and gerontology in medically underserved areas. *J Contin Educ Health Profs*. 2009;29(3):157-160.

49. Gooding HC, Ziniel S, Touloumtzis C, et al. Case-based teaching for interprofessional postgraduate trainees in adolescent health. *J Adolesc Health*. 2016;58(5):567-572.

50. Bonwell PB, Parsons PL, Best AM, Hise S. An interprofessional education approach to oral health care in the geriatric population. *Gerontol Geriatr Educ*. 2014;35(2):182-199.

51. Lundon K, Shupak R, Reeves S, Schneider R, McIlroy JH. The advanced clinician practitioner in arthritis care program: an interprofessional model for transfer of knowledge for advanced practice practitioners. *J Interprof Care*. 2009;23(2):1998-200.

52. Villarreal D, Restrepo MI, Healy J, et al. A model for increasing palliative care in the intensive care unit: enhancing interprofessional consultation rates and communication. *J Pain Symptom Manage*. 2011;42(5):676-679.

53. Robben S, Perry M, van Nieuwenhuijzen L, van Achterberg T, Rikkert MO, Schers H, Heinen M, Melis R. Impact of interprofessional education on collaboration, attitudes, skills, and behavior among primary care professionals. *J Continuing Educ Health Profs*. 2012;32(3):196-204.

54. Smith S, Karban K. Tutor experiences of developing an interprofessional learning program (ILP) in higher education. *Response*. 2008;4(1):1-13.

55. Howkins E, Bray J, eds. *Preparing for Interprofessional Teaching: Theory and Practice*. Oxford, United Kingdom: Radcliffe; 2008.

56. Freeth D, Hammick M, Reeves S, Koppel I, Barr H. 2005. *Effective Interprofessional Education: Development, Delivery and Evaluation*. Oxford, UK: Blackwell.

57. Simmons B, Egan-Lee E, Wagner SJ, Esdaile M, Baker L, Reeves S. Assessment of interprofessional learning: the design of an interprofessional objective structured clinical examination (iOSCE) approach. *J Interprof Care*. 2011;25:73-74.

58. Pien LC, Stiber M, Prelosky A, Colbert, CY. Interprofessional educator development. *Perspect Med Educ.* 2018;7(3):214-218. https://doi.org/10.1007/s40037-018-0418-9

59. Guraya SY, Barr H. The effectiveness of interprofessional education in healthcare: a systematic review and meta-analysis. *Kaohsiung J Med Sci.* 2018;34:160-165.

60. Shrader S, Farland MZ, Danielson J, Sicat B, Umland EM. A systematic review of assessment tools measuring interprofessional education outcomes relevant to pharmacy education. *Am J Pharm Educ.* 2017;81(6):119. doi:10.5688/ajpe816119

61. Ratka A, Zorek JA, Meyer SM. Overview of faculty development programs for interprofessional education. *Am J Pharm Educ.* 2017;81(5):96. doi:10.5688/ajpe81596

62. Chiu C, Zierler B, Brock D, Demiris G, Taibi D, Scott C. *Development and Validation of Performance Assessment Tools for Interprofessional Communication and Teamwork (PACT)* [dissertation]. Seattle: University of Washington; 2014.

63. Chiu C, Brock D, Abu-Rish E. Performance Assessment of Communication and Teamwork (PACT) tool set. Center for Interprofessional Education, Research, and Practice; University of Washington. http://collaborate.uw.edu/tools-and-curricula/tools-forevaluation/performance-assessment-of-communication-andteamwork-pact-t. Accessed May 5, 2018.

64. Hayward MF, Curran V, Curtis B, Schulz H, Murphy S. Reliability of the interprofessional collaborator assessment rubric (ICAR) in multi source feedback (MSF) with post-graduate medical residents. *BMC Med Educ.* 2014;14:1049.

65. Archibold D, Trumpower D, MacDonald C. Validation of the Interprofessional Collaborative Competency Attainment Survey (ICCAS). *J Interprof Care.* 2014;28:553-558.

66. Dow AW, DiazGranados D, Mazmania PE, Retchin SM. An exploratory study of an assessment tool derived from the competencies of the Interprofessional Education Collaborative. *J Interprof Care.* 2014;28(4):299-304.

67. Oliver D, Connelly J, Victor C, et al. Strategies to prevent falls and fractures in hospitals and care homes and effect of cognitive impairment. Systematic review and meta-analyses. *BMJ* 2007;334:82-7.

68. Curran V, Hollett A, Casimiro LM, Mccarthy P, Banfield V, Hall P, Lackie K, Oandasan I, Simmons B, Wagner S. Development and validation of the interprofessioanl collaborator assessment rubric (ICAR). *J Interprof Care.* 2011;25(5):339-344.

69. Keshmiri F, Ponzer S, Sohrabpour AA, Farahmand Sh, Shahi F, Bagheri-Hariri Sh, Soltani-Arabshahi K, Shirazi M, Masiello I. Contextualization and validation of the Interprofessional Collaborator Assessment Rubric (ICAR) through simulation: pilot investigation. *Med J Islam Repub Iran.* August 2016;(30):403.

70. Zorek J, Raehl C. Interprofessional education accreditation standards in the USA: a comparative analysis. *J Interprof Care.* 2013;27(2):123-130.

71. Health Professions Accreditors Collaborative (HPAC). *Guidance on Developing Quality Interprofessional Education for the Health Professions.* Chicago, IL: HPAC; 2019.

72. McCutcheon LRM, Whitcomb K, Cox CD, Klein MS, Burley H, Youngblood T, Raehl C. Interprofessional objective structured teaching exercise (iOSTE) to train preceptors. *Curr Pharm Teach Learn.* July 2017;9(4):605-615.

73. Congdon HB, Cate K. Development and integration of an interprofessional education (IPE) clinic visit flowsheet for health professions students. *J Interprof Educ Pract.* 2019;16:100249.

74. Walker SE, Cavallario JM, Welch Bacon CE, Bay RC, Van Lunen BL. Athletic training student application of interprofessional education during clinical education: a report

from the Athletic Training Clinical Education Network. Presented at: 2019 NATA Athletic Training Educators' Conference; February 15-17, 2019; Grapevine, TX. Abstract published in *Athl Train Educ J.* 2018;13(4):391-392.

75. Hudak NM, Melcher B, Strand de Oliveira J. Preceptors' perceptions of interprofessional practice, student interactions, and strategies for interprofessional education in clinical settings. *J Physician Assist Educ.* 2017;(4):214.

76. Zorek JA, Blaszczyk AT, Haase MR, Raehl CL. Practice Site Readiness for Interprofessional Education (PRIPE): instrument development and pilot study. *Curr Pharm Teach Learn.* 2014;6(1):32-40.

77. Parry, M, Utley, JJ, Shapiro, S, Podlog, S. (2019). Faculty perceptions of readiness to implement interprofessional education in athletic training. *Health Interprof Pract.* 3(4).

78. Shrader S, Zaudke J. Top ten best practices for interprofessional precepting. *J Interprof Educ Pract.* 2018;10:56-60.

79. Welsch LA, Rutledge C, Hoch JM. The modified Readiness for Interprofessional Learning Scale in currently practicing athletic trainers. *Athl Train Educ J.* 2017;(1):10.

80. Botma Y. Consensus on interprofessional facilitator capabilities. *J Interprof Care.* 2019;33(3):277-279.

81. Weiss KB, Passiment M, Riordan L, Wagner R for the National Collaborative for Improving the Clinical Learning Environment IP-CLE Report Work Group. Achieving the Optimal Interprofessional Clinical Learning Environment: Proceedings From an NCICLE Symposium. http://ncicle.org. Published January 18, 2019. doi:10.33385/NCICLE.0002

82. Hawkins R, Silvester JA, Passiment M, Riordan L, Weiss KB for the National Collaborative for Improving the Clinical Learning Environment IP-CLE Planning Group. *Envisioning the Optimal Interprofessional Clinical Learning Environment: Initial Findings From an October 2017 NCICLE Symposium.* http://ncicle.org. Published January 12, 2018.

Chapter 4

1. Bodenheimer T, Sinsky C. From Triple to Quadruple Aim: care of the patient requires care of the provider. *Ann Fam Med.* 2014;12(6):573-576.

2. Loversidge J, Demb, A. Faculty perceptions of key factors in interprofessional education. *J Interprof Care.* 2104;29(4):298-304.

3. Freeth, D, Reeves, S. Learning to work together: using the presage, process, product (3P) model to highlight decisions and possibilities. *J Interprof Care.* 2004;18(1):43-56.

4. Watkins K. Faculty development to support interprofessional education in healthcare professions: a realist approach. *J Interprof Care.* 2016;30(6):695-701.

5. Malechwanzi JM, Lei H, Wang L. Students' perceptions and faculty measured competencies in higher education. *Int J High Educ.* 2016;5(3):56-69.

6. Hall L, Zierler B. Interprofessional education and practice guide no. 1: developing faculty to effectively facilitate interprofessional education. *J Interprof Care.* 2015;29:3-7.

7. Ratka, A. Transition of pharmacy educators to faculty champions of interprofessional education. *Am J Pharm Educ.* 2013;77(7):136.

8. Institute of Medicine (IOM). *Health Professions Education: A Bridge to Quality.* Washington, DC: National Academies Press; 2003. https://doi.org/10.17226/10681

9. Institute of Medicine (IOM). *Crossing the Quality Chasm: A New Health System for the 21st Century.* Washington, DC: National Academic Press; 2001.

10. Dahlgren L, Gibbs D, Greenwalt S, Hahn L, Dietrich M. Getting it right from the start: an interprofessional orientation experience for graduate health sciences students, evaluating attitudes toward role. *OALib J*. 2018;5:1-15.

11. Lockeman KS, Appelbaum NP, Dow AW, Orr S, Huff TA, Hogan CJ, Queen BA. The effect of an interprofessional simulation-based education program on perceptions and stereotypes of nursing and medical students: a quasi-experimental study. *Nurse Educ Today*. 2017;58:32-37.

12. Horbar JD, Rogowski J, Plsek PE, et al. Collaborative quality improvement for neonatal intensive care. *Pediatrics*. 2001;107(1):14-22.

13. Dienst ER, Byl N. Evaluation of an educational program in health care teams. *J Community Health*. 1981;6(4):282.

14. Reeves S, Boet S, Zierler B, Kitto S. Interprofessional education and practice guide no. 3: evaluating interprofessional education. *J Interprof Care*. 2015;29(4):305-312.

15. Pham MT, Rajić A, Greig JD, Sargeant JM, Papadopoulos A, McEwen SA. A scoping review of scoping reviews: advancing the approach and enhancing the consistency. *Res Synth Methods*. 2014;5(4):371-385.

16. Reeves S, Fletcher S, Barr H, Birch I, Boet S, Davies N, McFadyen A, Rivera J, Kitto S. A BEME systematic review of the effects of interprofessional education: BEME Guide No. 39. *Med Teach*. 2016;38(7):656-668. doi:10.3109/0142159X.2016.1173663

17. Berwick DM, Nolan TW, Whittington J. The Triple Aim: care, health, and cost. *Health Aff*. 2008;27(3):759-769.

18. Haas JS, Cook EF, Puopolo AL, Burstin HR, Cleary PD, Brennan TA. Is the professional satisfaction of general internists associated with patient satisfaction? *J Gen Intern Med*. 2000;15(2):122-128.

19. McHugh MD, Kutney-Lee A, Cimiotti JP, Sloane DM, Aiken LH. Nurses' widespread job dissatisfaction, burnout, and frustration with health benefits signal problems for patient care. *Health Aff (Millwood)*. 2011;30(2):202-210.

20. Williams ES, Skinner AC. Outcomes of physician job satisfaction: a narrative review, implications, and directions for future research. *Health Care Manage Rev*. 2003;28(2):119-139.

21. DiMatteo MR, Sherbourne CD, Hays RD, et al. Physicians' characteristics influence patients' adherence to medical treatment: results from the Medical Outcomes Study. *Health Psychol*. 1993;12(2):93-102.

22. Kushnir T, Greenberg D, Madjar N, Hadari I, Yermiahu Y, Bachner YG. Is burnout associated with referral rates among primary care physicians in community clinics? *Fam Pract*. 2014;31(1):44-50.

23. Homeyer S, Hoffmann W, Hingst P, Oppermann RF, Dreier-Wolfgramm A. Effects of interprofessional education for medical and nursing students: enablers, barriers and expectations for optimizing future interprofessional collaboration—a qualitative study. *BMC Nurs*. 2018;17:13. doi:10.1186/s12912-018-0279-x

24. Lash, DB, Barnett MJ, Parekh N, Shieh A, Louie MC, Tang TT. Perceived benefits and challenges of interprofessional education based on a multidisciplinary faculty member survey. *Am J Pharm Educ*. 2014;78(10):Article 180.

25. Morphet J, Hood, K, Cant, R, Baulch, J, Gilbee, A, Sandry, K. Teaching teamwork: an evaluation of an interprofessional training ward placement for healthcare students. *Adv Med Educ Pract*. 2014;5:197-204.

26. Bodenheimer T, Willard-Grace R, Ghorob A. Expanding the roles of medical assistants: who does what in primary care? *JAMA Intern Med*. 2014;174(7):1025-1026.

27. Bodenheimer TS, Smith MD. Primary care: proposed solutions to the physician shortage without training more physicians. *Health Aff (Millwood)*. 2013;32(11):1881-1886.

28. Friedberg MW, Chen PG, Van Busum KR, et al. Factors affecting physician professional satisfaction and their implications for patient care, health systems and health policy. www.rand.org/content/dam/rand/pubs/research_reports/ RR400/ RR439/RAND_RR439.pdf. Published 2013. Accessed March 25, 2019.

29. IOM (Institute of Medicine). Measuring the impact of interprofessional education on collaborative practice and patient outcomes. Washington, DC: National Academies Press; 2015.

30. Riskiyana R, Claramita M, Rahayu G. Objectively measured interprofessional education outcome and factors that enhance program effectiveness: a systematic review. *Nurse Educ Today*. July 2018;66:73-78.

31. Shrader S, Farland MZ, Danielson J, Sicat B, Umland EM. A systematic review of assessment tools measuring interprofessional education outcomes relevant to pharmacy education. *Am J Pharm Educ*. 2017;81(6):119. doi:10.5688/ajpe816119

32. Baker C, Pulling C, McGraw R, Dagnone JD, Hopkins-Rosseel D, Medves J. Simulation in interprofessional education for patient-centered collaborative care. *J Adv Nurs*. 2008;64(4):372-379.

33. MacDonald MB, Bally JM, Ferguson LM, Lee Murray B, Fowler-Kerry SE, Anonson JMS. Knowledge of the professional role of others: a key interprofessional competency. *Nurse Educ Pract*. 2010;10:238-242.

34. McNeil KA, Mitchell RJ, Parker, V. Interprofessional practice and professional identity threat. *Health Sociol Rev*. 2013;22(3):291-307.

35. Roberts LD, Davis MC, Radley-Crabb HG, Broughton M. Perceived relevance mediates the relationship between professional identity and attitudes toward interprofessional education in first-year university students. *J Interprof Care*. 2018;32(1):33-40.

36. Zamjahn JB, Beyer EO, Alig KL, Mercante DE, Carter KL, Gunaldo TP. Increasing awareness of the roles, knowledge, and skills of respiratory therapists through an interprofessional education experience. *Resp Care*. 2018;63(5):510-518.

37. Michalec, B, Giordano, C, Pugh, B, Arenson, C, Speakman, E. Health professions students' perceptions of their IPE program. *J Allied Health*. 2017;46(1):10-20.

38. Soubra L, Badr SBY, Zahran EM, Aboul-Seoud M. Effect of interprofessional education on role clarification and patient care planning by health professions students. *Health Prof Educ*. 2018;4:317-328.

39. Stull CL, Blue CM. Examining the influence of professional identity formation on the attitudes of students towards interprofessional collaboration. *J Interprof Care*. 2016;30(1):90-96.

40. Granheim BM, Shaw JM, Mansah M. The use of interprofessional learning and simulation in undergraduate nursing programs to address interprofessional communication and collaboration: an integrative review of the literature. *Nurs Educ Today*. 2018;62:118-127.

41. Vermeir P, Vandijck D, Degroote S, Peleman R, Verhaeghe R, Mortier EÉ, Vogelaers D. Communication in healthcare: a narrative review of the literature and practical recommendations. *Int J Clin Pract*. 2015;69(11):1257-1267.

42. McGehee WF, Dunleavy K, Blue AV, Stetten NE, Black EW. Physical interprofessional learning experience. *J Phys Ther Educ*. 2018;32(1):70-76.

43. Dicker R, Garcia M, Kelly A, Modabber P, O'Farrell A, Pond A, Pond N, Mulrooney HM. Student perceptions of quality in higher education: effect of year of study, gender and ethnicity. *New Dir Teach Phys Sci*. 2017;12(1):1-14.

44. Radovan M, Makovec D. Relations between students' motivation, and perceptions of the learning environment. *Cent Educ Pol Stud J*. 2015;5(2):115-138.

45. Liaw SY, Zhou WT, Lau TC, Siau C, Chan SW. An interprofessional communication training using simulation to enhance safe care for a deteriorating patient. *Nurse Educ Today*. 2014;34:259-264. doi:10.1016/j.nedt.2013.02.019

46. Allen IE, Seaman J. Digital learning compass: distance education enrollment report 2017. Copyright © 2017 by Babson Survey Research Group, e-Literate, and WCET.

47. McKee N, D'Eon M, Trinder K. Problem-based learning for interprofessional education: evidence from an inter-professional PBL module on palliative care. *Can Med Educ J*. 2013;4(1):35-48.

48. Kyriakoulis K, Patelarou A, Laliotis A, Wan AC, Maralliotakis M, Tsiou C, Patelarou E. Educational strategies for teaching evidence-based practice in undergraduate health students: systematic review. *J Educ Eval Health Prof*. 2016;13(34):1-10.

49. Chen AK, Dennehy C, Fitzsimmons A, Hyde S, Lee K, Rivera J, Shunk R, Warmsley M. Teaching interprofessional collaborative care skills using a blended learning approach. *J Interprof Educ Pract*. 2017;8:86-90.

50. Lo V, Wu RC, Morra D, Lee L, Reeves S. The use of smartphones in general and internal medicine units: a boon or a bane to the promotion of interprofessional collaboration? *J Interprof Care*. 2012;26(4):276-282.

51. McCutcheon LR, Alzghari SK, Lee YR, Long WG, Marquez R. Interprofessional education and distance education: a review and appraisal of the current literature. *Curr Pharm Teach Learn*. 2017;9(4):729-736.

52. Watts, L. Synchronous and asynchronous communication in distance learning: a review of the literature. *Q Rev Distance Educ*. 2016;17(1):23-32.

53. Interprofessional Education Collaborative (IPEC). *Core Competencies for Interprofessional Collaborative Practice: 2016 Update*. Washington, DC: IPEC; 2016.

54. World Health Organization (WHO). Framework for Action on Interprofessional Education and Collaborative Practice. Geneva, Switzerland: WHO; 2010.

55. Walmsley L, Fortune M, Brown A. Experiential interprofessional education for medical students at a regional medical campus. *Can Med Educ J*. 2018;9(1):e59-e67.

56. Pollard K, Miers ME, Gilchrist M. Second year scepticism: pre-qualifying health and social care students' midpoint self-assessment, attitudes and perceptions concerning interprofessional learning and working. *J Interprof Care*. 2005;19(3):251-268.

57. Gore, T, Thomson, W. Use of simulation in undergraduate and graduate education. *Sim Nurs Educ*. 2016;27(1):86-95.

58. INACSL Standards Committee. INACSL standards of best practice: Simulation^SM facilitation. *Clin Sim Nurs*, December 2016;12(S):S16-S20.

59. Ryall T, Judd BK, Gordon CJ. Simulation-based assessments in health professional education: a systematic review. *J Multidiscip Healthc*. 2016;1:69-82.

60. Curl ED, Smith S, Chisholm L, McGee LA, Das K. Effectiveness of integrated simulation and clinical experiences compared to traditional clinical experiences for nursing students. *Nurs Educ Perspect*. 2016;37(2):72-77.

61. Kim J, Park J, Shin S. Effectiveness of simulation-based nursing education depending on fidelity: a meta-analysis. *BMC Med Educ*. 2016;16:152.

62. National Council of State Boards of Nursing (NCSBN). The NCSBN National Simulation Study: a longitudinal, randomized, controlled study replacing

clinical hours with simulation in prelicensure nursing education. *J Nurs Regul*. 2014;5(suppl):S3-S40.

63. McDougall, EM. Simulation in education for healthcare professionals. *BC Med J*. 2015;57(10):444-448.

64. Evans S, Sønderlund A, Tooley G. Effectiveness of online interprofessional education in improving students' attitudes and knowledge associated with interprofessional practice. *Focus Health Prof Educ*. 2014;14(2):12-20.

65. Evan SM, Ward C, Reeves S. An exploration of teaching presence in online interprofessional education facilitation. *Med Teach*. 2017;39(7):773-779.

66. Dunleavy K, Galen S, Reid K, Dhar JP, DiZazzo-Miller R. Impact of interprofessional peer teaching on physical and occupational therapy student's professional role identity. *J Interprof Educ Pract*. 2017;6:1-5.

67. Eggenberger T, Sherman RO, Keller K. Creating high-performance interprofessional teams. *Am Nurse Today*. 2014;9(11):12-14.

68. Aveling EL, Stone J, Sundt T, Wright C, Gino F, Singer S. Factors influencing team behaviors in surgery: a qualitative study to inform teamwork interventions. *Ann Thorac Surg*. 2018;106:115-120.

69. Goto M, Haruta J, Oishi A, Yoshida K, Yoshimi K, Takemura Y, Yoshimoto H. A cross-section survey of interprofessional education across 13 healthcare professions in Japan. *TAPS*. 2018;3(2):37-45.

70. Shiyanbola OO, Randall B, Lammers C, Hegge KA, Anderson M. Impact of an interprofessional diabetes education model on patient health outcomes: a longitudinal study. *J Res Interprof Pract Educ*. 2014;4(2):1-21.

71. Clifton M, Dale C, Bradshaw C. *The Impact and Effectiveness of Interprofessional Education in Primary Care: An RCN Literature Review*. London, England: Royal College of Nursing; 2006.

72. Hammick M, Freeth D, Koppel I, Reeves S, Barr H. A best evidence systematic review of interprofessional education. *Med Teach*. 2007;29(8):735-751.

73. Thannhauser J, Russell-Mayhew S, Scott C. Measures of interprofessional education and collaboration. *J Interprof Care*. 2010;24(4):336-349.

74. Ralyea, CM. *For Labor and Delivery Staff, How Does the Implementation of TeamSTEPPS Compared to Current Practice Impact Quality Indicators Over a Six-Month Period?* [dissertation]. Minneapolis: Capella University; 2013.

75. Rotz ME, Dueñas GG, Zanoni A, Grover AB. Designing and evaluating an interprofessional experiential course involving medical and pharmacy students. *Am J Pharm Educ*. 2016;80:85.

76. Wilhelmsson M, Pelling S, Ludvigsson J, Hammar M, Dahlgren LO, Faresjo T. Twenty years experiences of interprofessional education in Linkoping—ground-breaking and sustainable. *J Interprof Care*. 2009;23(2):121-133. doi:10.1080/13561820902728984

77. Zaudke JK, Chestnut C, Paolo A, Shrader S. The impact of an interprofessional practice experience on student behaviors related to interprofessional communication and teamwork. *J Interprof Educ Pract*. 2016;4:9-13.

78. Brewer ML, Stewart-Wynne EG. An Australian hospital-based student training ward delivering safe, client-centred care while developing students' interprofessional practice capabilities. *J Interprof Care*. 2013;27(6):482-488.

79. Hallin K, Henriksson P, Dalén N, Kiessling A. Effects of interprofessional education on patient perceived quality of care. *Med Teach*. 2011;33(1):e22-e26.

80. Kent F, Keating J. Patient outcomes from a student-led interprofessional clinic in primary care. *J Interprof Care*. 2013;27(4):336-338.

81. West M, Boshoff K, Stewart H. A qualitative exploration of the characteristics and practices of interdisciplinary collaboration. *S Afr J Occup Ther*. 2016;46(3):27-34.

82. Shirey MR, White-Williams C, Hites L. Integration of authentic leadership lens for building high performing interprofessional collaborative practice teams. *Nurs Adm Q*. 2019;43(2):101-112.

83. Bates SM, Mellin E, Paluta LM, Anderson-Butcher D, Vogeler M, Sterling K. Examining the influence of interprofessional team collaboration on student-level outcomes though school-community partnerships. *Child School*. 2019;(41)2:111-122.

84. Brashers V, Haizlip J, Owen JA. The ASPIRE model: grounding the IPEC core competencies for IPCP with a foundational framework. *J Interprof Care*. 2019. https://doi.org/10.1080/13561820.2019.1624513

85. McCutcheon LRM, Whitcomb K, Cox CD, Klein MS, Burley H, Youngblood T, Raehl C. Interprofessional objective structured teaching exercise (iOSTE) to train preceptors. *Curr Pharm Teach Learn*. 2017;9(4):605-615.

86. Congdon HB, Cate K. Development and integration of an interprofessional education (IPE) clinic visit flowsheet for health professions students. *J Interprof Educ Pract*. 2019;16:100249.

87. Walker SE, Cavallario JM, Welch Bacon CE, Bay RC, Van Lunen BL. Athletic training student application of interprofessional education during clinical education: a report from the Athletic Training Clinical Education Network. Presented at 2019 NATA Athletic Training Educators' Conference; February 15-17, 2019; Grapevine, TX. Abstract published in *Athl Train Educ J*. 2018;13(4):391-392.

88. Hudak NM, Melcher B, Strand de Oliveira J. Preceptors' perceptions of interprofessional practice, student interactions, and strategies for interprofessional education in clinical settings. *J Physician Assist Educ*. 2017;4:214.

89. Zorek JA, Blaszczyk AT, Haase MR, Raehl CL. Practice Site Readiness for Interprofessional Education (PRIPE): instrument development and pilot study. *Curr Pharm Teach Learn*. 2014;6(1):32-40.

90. Sick B, Radosevich DM, Pittenger AL, Brandt B. Development and validation of a tool to assess the readiness of a clinical teaching site for interprofessional education (InSITE). *J Interprof Care*. 2019;11:1-11. DOI:10.1080/13561820.2019.1569600

91. Chiu C. Development and Validation of Performance Assessment Tools for Interprofessional Communication and Teamwork (PACT). 2014.

92. Hawk C, Buckwalter K, Byrd L, Cigelman S, Dorfman L, Ferguson K. Health professions students' perceptions of interprofessional relationships. *Acad Med*. 2002;77:354-357. pmid:11953306

93. Heinemann GD, Schmitt MH, Farrell MP, Brallier SA. Development of an attitudes toward health care teams scale. *Eval Health Prof*. 1999;22(1):123-142.

94. Curran V R, Sharpe D, Forristall J, Flynn K. Attitudes of health sciences students towards interprofessional teamwork and education. *Learning in Health and Social Care*. 2008;7(3):146-156.

95. Curran VR, Heath O, Kearney A, Button P. Evaluation of an interprofessional collaboration workshop for post-graduate residents, nursing and allied health professionals. *J Interprof Care*. 2010;24(3):315-318.

96. Olander E, Coates R, Brook J, Ayers S, Salmon D. A multi-method evaluation of interprofessional education for healthcare professionals caring for women during and after pregnancy. *J Interprof Care*. 2018;32(4):509-512. DOI: 10.1080/13561820.2018.1437124

97. Seaman K, Saunders R, Dugmore H, Tobin C, Singer R, Lake F. Shifts in nursing and medical student's attitudes, beliefs and behaviours about interprofessional work: An interprofessional placement in ambulatory care. *J Clin Nurs*. 2018;27(15). DOI: 10.1111/jocn.14506

98. Schack-Dugré J. Efficacy of online low-fidelity interprofessional education simulation. 2019.

99. Shipman SA, Sinsky CA. Expanding primary care capacity by reducing waste and improving the efficiency of care. *Health Aff (Millwood)*. 2013;32(11):1990-1997.

100. Pfaff K, Baxter P, Jack S, Ploeg J. An integrative review of the factors influencing new graduate nurse engagement in interprofessional collaboration. *J Adv Nurs*. 2014;70(1):4-20. doi: 10.1111/jan.12195.

101. Arenson C, Umland E, Collins L, Kern S, Hewston LA, Jerpbak C, Antony R, Rose M, Lyons K. The health mentors program: three years experience with longitudinal, patient-centered interprofessional education. *J Interprof Care*. 2015;29(2):138-143. DOI: 10.3109/13561820.2014.944257.

102. Bates S, Mellin E, Paluta L, Anderson-Butcher D, Vogeler M, Sterling K. Examining the influence of interprofessional team collaboration on student-level outcomes through school-community partnerships. *Children & Schools*. 2019;41(2):111-122.

103. Berg B, Wong L, Vincent D. Technology-enabled interprofessional education for nursing and medical students: A pilot study. *J Interprof Care*. 2010;24:601-604. doi: https://doi.org/10.3109/13561820903373194

104. Wellmon R, Gilin B, Knauss L, Linn M I. Changes in student attitudes toward interprofessional learning and collaboration arising from a case-based educational experience. *J Allied Health*. 2012:41(1):26-34.

105. Zorek J, Raehl C. Interprofessional education accreditation standards in the USA: a comparative analysis. *J Interprof Care*. 2013;27(2):123-130.

106. Cooke S, Chew G, Boggis C, Wakefield A. I never realised that doctors were into feelings too: changing student perceptions through interprofessional education. *Learn Health Soc Care*. 2003;2:137-146.

107. Ketola E, Sipila R, Makela M, Klockars M. Quality improvement programme for cardiovascular disease risk factor recording in primary care. *Qual Health Care*. 2000;9:175-180.

108. Morin C, Desrosiers J, Gaboury I. Enablers and barriers to the development of interprofessional collaboration between physicians and osteopaths: A mixed methods study. *J Interprof Care*. 2018;32:463-472.

109. Shafer MB, Tebb KP, Pantell RH, et al. Effect of a clinical practice improvement intervention on chlamydial screening among adolescent girls. *JAMA*. 2002;288(22):2846-2852. doi:10.1001/jama.288.22.2846

110. Shirey MR, White-Williams C, Hites L. Integration of authentic leadership lens for building high performing interprofessional collaborative practice teams. *Nurs Adm Q*. 2019;43(2):101-112.

111. Magnan S, Solberg LI, Kottke TE, Nelson AF, Amundson GM, Richards S, Reed MK. IMPROVE: bridge over troubled waters. *Jt Comm J Qual Imporv*. 1998;24(10): 566-578.

112. Kilminster S, Roberts T. Standard setting for OSCEs: trial of borderline approach. *Adv Health Sci Educ Theory Pract*. 2008;9(3):201-209.

113. Morey JC, Simon R, Jay GD, Wears RL, Salisbury M, Dukes KA, Berns SD. Error reduction and performance improvement in the emergency department through formal teamwork training: evaluation results of the MedTeams project. *Health Serv Res*. 2002;37(6):1553-1581.

114. Mu K, Chao CC, Jensen GM, Royeen CB. Effects of interprofessional rural training on students' perceptions of interprofessional health care services. *J Allied Health.* 2004;33(2):125-131.

115. Pollard KC, Miers ME, Gilchrist M. Collaborative learning for collaborative working? Initial findings from a longitudinal study of health and social care students. *Health Soc Care Community.* 2004;12(4):346-358.

116. Baker DP, Krokos KJ, Amodeo AM. TeamSTEPPS Teamwork Attitudes Questionnaire (T-TAQ) Manual. 2008. Washington, DC: American Institutes for Research.

117. Parsell G, Bligh J. The development of a questionnaire to assess the readiness of health care students for interprofessional learning (RIPLS). *Med Educ.* 1999;33(2):95-100.

118. Hawk C, Buckwalter K, Byrd L, Cigelman S, Dorfman L, Ferguson K. Health professions students' perceptions of interprofessional relationships. *Acad Med.* 2002;77(4):354-357.

119. Heinemann GD, Schmitt MH, Farrell MP, Brallier SA. Development of an attitudes toward health care teams scale. *Eval Health Prof.* 1999;22(1):123-142.

120. Curran V R, Sharpe D, Forristall J. Attitudes of health sciences faculty members towards interprofessional teamwork and education. *Med Educ.* 2007;41(9):892-896.

121. Zorek JA, Fike DS, Eickhoff JC, Engle JA, MacLaughlin EJ, Dominguez DG, Seibert CS. Refinement and validation of the student perceptions of physician-pharmacist interprofessional clinical education instrument. *Am J Pharm Educ.* 2016;80(3):1-8.

122. King G, Orchard C, Khalili H, Avery L. Refinement of the Interprofessional Socialization and Valuing Scale (ISVS-21) and development of 9-item equivalent versions. *J Contin Educ Health Prof.* 2016;36(3):171-177.

123. Orchard CA, King GA, Khalili H, Bezzina MB. Assessment of interprofessional team collaboration scale (AITCS): Development and testing of the instrument. *J Contin Educ Health Prof.* 2012;32(1):58-67.

124. Grymonpre R, van Ineveld C, Nelson M, Jensen F, De Jaeger A, Sullivan T, Weinberg L, Swinamer J, Booth A. See it – Do it – Learn it: Learning interprofessional collaboration in the clinical context. *J Res Interprof Pract Educ.* 2010;1(2):127-144.

125. Curran V, Hollett A, Casimiro LM, Mccarthy P, Banfield V, Hall P, Lackie K, Oandasan I, Simmons B, Wagner S. Development and validation of the interprofessional collaborator assessment rubric (ICAR). *J Interprof Care.* 2011;25(5):339-344.

126. Archibald D, Trumpower D, MacDonald CJ. Validation of the interprofessional collaborative competency attainment survey (ICCAS). *J Interprof Care.* 2014;28(6):553-558. doi: 10.3109/13561820.2014.917407

127. Kenaszchuk C, Reeves S, Nicholas D, Zwarenstein M. Validity and reliability of a multiple-group measurement scale for interprofessional collaboration. *BMC Health Serv Res.* 2010;10:83. doi: 10.1186/1472-6963-10-83

128. Dow AW, DiazGranados D, Mazmanian PE, Retchin SM. An exploratory study of an assessment tool derived from the competencies of the Interprofessional Education Collaborative. *J Interprof Care.* 2014;28(4):299-304. doi: 10.3109/13561820.2014.891573

129. Temkin-Greener H, Gross D, Kunitz SJ, Mukamel D. Measuring interdisciplinary team performance in a long-term care setting. *Medical Care.* 2004;42(5):472-481.

130. Careau E, Vincent C, Swaine BR. Observed interprofessional collaboration (OIPC) during interdisciplinary team meetings: Development and validation of a tool in a rehabilitation setting. *J Res Interprof Pract Educ.* 2014;4(1).

131. Chiu CJ. Development and validation of performance assessment tools for interprofessional communication and teamwork (PACT). 2014. Unpublished doctoral dissertation, University of Washington.

132. Parker Oliver D, Wittenberg-Lyles EM, Day M. Measuring interdisciplinary perceptions of collaboration on hospice teams. *Am J Hosp Palliat Care.* 2007;24(1):49-53.

133. Upenieks VV, Lee EA, Flanagan ME, Doebbeling BN. Healthcare Team Vitality Instrument (HTVI): Developing a tool assessing healthcare team functioning. *J Adv Nurs.* 2019;66(1):168-176.

134. Cartwright J, Franklin D, Forman D, Freegard H. Promoting collaborative dementia care via online interprofessional education. *Australas J Ageing.* 2013;34(2):88-94.

135. Coleman MT, Roberts K, Wulff D, van Zyl R, Newton K. Interprofessional ambulatory primary care practice-based educational program. *J Interprof Care.* 2008;22(1): 69-84.

136. Curran VR, Sharpe D, Flynn K, Button P. A longitudinal study of the effect of an interprofessional education curriculum on student satisfaction and attitudes towards interprofessional teamwork and education. *J Interprof Care.* 2010;24(1):41-52.

137. Dallaghan GLB, Hultquist TB, Nickol D, Collier D, Geske J. Attitudes toward interprofessional education improve over time. *J Interprof Educ Pract.* 2018;13:24-26.

138. Iachini AL, DeHart DD, Browne T, Dunn BL, Blake EW, Blake C. Examining collaborative leadership through interprofessional education: findings from a mixed methods study. *J Interprof Care.* 2019;33(2):235-242.

139. Kenaszchuk C, Rykhoff M, Collins L, McPhail S, van Soeren M. Positive and null effects of interprofessional education on attitudes toward interprofessional learning and collaboration. *Adv Health Sci Educ Theory Pract.* 2012;17(5):651-669.

140. McFadyen AK, Webster VS, Maclaren WM, O'Neill MA. Interprofessional attitudes and perceptions: Results from a longitudinal controlled trial of pre-registration health and social care students in Scotland. *J Interprof Care.* 2010;24(5):549-564.

141. McLeod D, Curran J, Dumont S, White M, Charles G. The Interprofessional Psychosocial Oncology Distance Education (IPODE) project: perceived outcomes of an approach to healthcare professional education. *J Interprof Care.* 2014;28(3):254-259.

142. Packard K, Ryan-Haddad A, Monaghan MS, Doll J, Qi Y. Application of validated instruments to assess university-wide interprofessional service-learning experiences. *J Interprof Educ Pract.* 2016;4:69-75.

143. Pollard KC, Miers ME. From students to professionals: Results of a longitudinal study of attitudes to pre-qualifying collaborative learning and working in health and social care in the United Kingdom. *J Interprof Care.* 2008;22(4):399-416.

144. Pollard KC, Miers ME, Rickaby C. "Oh why didn't I take more notice?" Professionals' views and perceptions of pre-qualifying preparation for interprofessional working in practice. *J Interprof Care.* 2012;26(5):355-361.

145. Quesnelle KM, Bright DR, Salvati LA. Interprofessional education through a telehealth team based learning exercise focused on pharmacogenomics. *Curr Pharm Teach Learn.* 2018;10(8):1062-1069.

146. Rens L, Joosten A. Investigating the experiences in a school-based occupational therapy program to inform community-based paediatric occupational therapy practice. *Aust Occup Ther J.* 2014;61(3):148-158.

147. Shoemaker MJ, de Voest M, Booth A, Meny L, Victor J. A virtual patient educational activity to improve interprofessional competencies: a randomized trial. *J Interprof Care.* 2015;29(4):395-397.

148. Shrader S, Kostoff M, Shin T, Heble A, Kempin B, Miller A, Patykiewicz N. Using communication technology to enhance interprofessional education simulations. *Am J Pharm Educ*. 2016;80(1):13.

149. Solomon P, Geddes EL. An interprofessional e-learning module on health care ethics. *J Interprof Care*. 2018;24(3):311-314.

150. Sytsma TT, Haller EP, Youdas JW, Krause DA, Hellyer NJ, Pawlina W, Lachman N. Long-term effect of a short interprofessional education interaction between medical and physical therapy students. *Anat Sci Educ*. 2015;8(4):317-323.

151. Zanotti R, Sartor G, Canova C. Effectiveness of interprofessional education by on-field training for medical students, with a pre-post design. *BMC Med Educ*. 2015;15(1):121.

152. Wilhelmsson M, Svensson A, Timpka T, Faresjö T. Nurses' views of interprofessional education and collaboration: A comparative study of recent graduates from three universities. *J Interprof Care*. 213;27(2):155-160.

153. Dachtyl SA, Morales P. A collaborative model for return to academics after concussion: athletic training and speech-language pathology. *Am J Speech Lang Pathol*. 2017;26(3):716-728.

154. Reeves S, Freeth D. The London training ward: an innovative interprofessional learning initiative. *J Interprof Care*. 2002;16(1):41-52.

155. Van Eeghen CO, Littenberg B, Kessler R. Chronic care coordination by integrating care through a team-based, population-driven approach: a case study. *Transl Behav Med*. 2018;8(3):468-480.

Chapter 5

1. O'Daniel M, Rosenstein AH, Hughes RG. Professional communication and team collaboration. In: Hughes RG, ed. *Patient Safety and Quality: An Evidence-Based Handbook for Nurses*. Vol. 2. Rockville, MD: Agency for Healthcare Research and Quality; 2008:271-284. www.ncbi.nlm.nih.gov/books/NBK2637/pdf/Bookshelf_NBK2637.pdf. Accessed November 14, 2018.

2. Reeves S, Pelone F, Harrison R, Goldman J, Zwarenstein M. Interprofessional collaboration to improve professional practice and healthcare outcomes. *Cochrane Database Syst Rev*. 2017;6:CD000072. doi:10.1002/14651858.CD000072.pub3

3. Institute of Medicine (IOM). *Measuring the Impact of Interprofessional Education on Collaborative Practice and Patient Outcomes*. Washington, DC: National Academies Press; 2015. https://doi.org/10.17226/21726

4. Leonard M, Graham S, Bonacum D. The human factor: the critical importance of effective teamwork and communication in providing safe care. *Qual Saf Health Care*. 2004;13(suppl 1):i85-i90. doi:10.1136/qshc.2004.010033

5. Reeves S, Fletcher S, Barr H, Birch I, Boet S, Davies N, McFadyen A, Rivera J, Kitto S. A BEME systematic review of the effects of interprofessional education: BEME Guide No. 39. *Med Teach*. 2016;38(7):656-668. doi:10.3109/0142159X.2016.1173663

6. Reeves S, Palaganas J, Zierler B. An updated synthesis of review evidence of interprofessional education. *J Allied Health*. 2017;46(1):56-61.

7. Guraya SY, Hugh B. The effectiveness of interprofessional education in healthcare: a systematic review and meta-analysis. *Kaohsiung J Med Sci*. 2017;34(3):160-165.

8. World Health Organization (WHO). Framework for Action on Interprofessional Education and Collaborative Practice. Geneva, Switzerland: WHO; 2010.

9. Sexton M, Baessler M. Interprofessional collaborative practice. *J Cont Educ Nurs*. 2016;4:156-157.

10. Almost A, Wolff AC, Stewart-Pyne A, McCormick LG, Strachan D, D'Souza C. Managing and mitigating conflict in healthcare teams: an integrative review. *J Adv Nurs.* 2016;72(7):1490-1505.

11. Chen A. *Collaboration and Communication in Healthcare: Principles of Interprofessional Practice. Segment 1: Conflict in Health Care Setting* [video]. YouTube. www.youtube.com/watch?v=SKuEsaoB9jg&list=PLY1lnohv0ZTOeJJJe2b-0Lgss_KDvCaUS&index=2. Published June 9, 2016. Accessed August 6, 2018.

12. Edmondson AC, Harvey J. Cross-boundary teaming for innovation: integrating research on teams and knowledge in organizations. *Hum Resour Manag Rev.* December 2018;347-360.

13. Glossary. Interprofessional Professionalism Collaborative (IPC) website. www.interprofessionalprofessionalism.org/uploads/1/8/8/6/1886419/glossary_ipc_terms_08_2011.pdf. Published August 3, 2011. Accessed November 12, 2018.

14. Frost JS, Hammer DP, Nunez LM, et al. The intersection of professionalism and interprofessional care: development and initial testing of the Interprofessional Professionalism Assessment (IPA). *J Interprof Care.* September 2018;1-15. doi:10.1080/13561820.2018.1515733

15. Schein EH. *Helping: How to Offer, Give, and Receive Help.* Oakland, CA: Berrett-Koehler Publishers; 2009.

16. Edmondson AC, Lei Z. Psychological safety: the history, renaissance, and future of interpersonal construct. *Annu Rev Organ Psych.* 2014;1:23-43. doi:10.1146/annurev-orgpsych-031413-091305

17. Leggat SG. Effective healthcare teams require effective team members: defining teamwork competencies. *BMC Health Serv Res.* 2007;7:17. doi:10.1186/1472-6963-7-17

18. Tuckman BW, Jensen MA. Stages of small-group development revisited. *Group Facil.* 2010;10:43-48.

19. Brooks Automation. Supplier training: 8D problem solving approach. www.brooks.com/my-brooks/suppliers/~/media/Files/Suppliers/Documents/5_Why_Root_Cause_Corrective_Actions.pdf. Published 2013. Accessed November 14, 2018.

20. ERC. Team Oriented Problem Solving (TOPS) training. www.yourerc.com/training/team-oriented-problem-solving. Published 2018. Accessed November 14, 2018.

21. Graban M. *Lean Hospitals: Improving Quality, Patient Safety, and Employee Engagement.* 2nd ed. Boca Raton, FL: CRC Press; 2012.

22. Boslaugh, SE. *Six Sigma.* Hackensack, NJ: Salem Press Encyclopedia; 2013.

23. Layne DM, Nemeth LS, Mueller M, Martin M. Negative behaviors among healthcare professionals: relationship with patient safety culture. *Healthcare.* 2019;7(23):1-11. doi:10.3390/healthcare7010023

24. O'Leary KJ, Johnson JK, Manojlovich M, Goldstein JD, Lee J, Williams MV. Redesigning systems to improve teamwork and quality for hospitalized patients (RESET): study protocol evaluating the effect of mentored implementation to redesign clinical microsystems. *BMC Health Serv Res.* 2019;19(293):1-11. http://doi.org/10.1186/s12913-019-4116-z

Chapter 6

1. Edmondson A. *Teaming: How Organizations Learn, Innovate, and Compete in the Knowledge Economy.* Hoboken, NJ: Jossey-Bass Pfeiffer; 2014.

2. Cohen SG, Bailey DR. What makes teams work: group effectiveness research from the shop floor to the executive suite. *J Manag.* 1997;23(4):238-290.

3. Berwick DM, Nolan TW, Whittington J. The Triple Aim: care, health, and cost. *Health Aff.* 2008;27(3):759-769.

4. Nancarrow SA, Booth A, Ariss S, Smith T, Enderby P, Roots A. Ten principles of good interdisciplinary team work. *Hum Resour Health.* 2013;11:19.

5. Interprofessional Education Collaborative (IPEC) Expert Panel. *Core Competencies for Interprofessional Collaborative Practice: Report of an Expert Panel.* Washington, DC: IPEC; 2011.

6. Committee on the Health Professions Education of the National Academy of Medicine. *Health Professions Education: A Bridge to Quality.* Washington, DC: National Academies Press; 2003.

7. Vega CP, Bernard A. Interprofessional collaboration to improve health care: an introduction. www.medscape.org/viewarticle/857823. Published 2016. Accessed November 18, 2018.

8. World Health Organization (WHO). Framework for Action on Interprofessional Education and Collaborative Practice. http://whqlibdoc.who.int/hq/2010/WHO_HRH_HPN_10.3_eng.pdf. Published 2010. Accessed November 18, 2018.

9. Kohn LT, Corrigan JM, Donaldson MS, eds. *To Err Is Human. Building a Safer Health System.* Washington, DC: National Academy Press; 2000.

10. Joint Commission. Human factors analysis in patient safety systems. www.jointcommission.org/assets/1/6/HumanFactorsThe_Source.pdf. Published 2015. Accessed November 18, 2018.

11. Brock D, Abu-Rish E, Chiu CR, et al. Interprofessional education in team communication: working together to improve patient safety. *BMJ Qual Saf.* 2013;22(5):414-423.

12. Ulrich B, Crider NM. Using teams to improve outcomes and performance. *Nephrol Nurs J.* 2017;44(2):141-151.

13. Agency for Healthcare Research and Quality (AHRQ). Team structure. www.ahrq.gov/sites/default/files/wysiwyg/professionals/education/curriculum-tools/teamstepps/instructor/fundamentals/module2/igteamstruct.pdf. Published 2017. Accessed November 18, 2018.

14. Janus I. *Group Think.* Boston, MA: Houghton Mifflin; 1982.

15. Bird AM. Team structure and success as related to cohesiveness and leadership. *J Soc Psychol.* 1977;103:217-233.

16. Urban JM, Bowers CA, Monday SD, Morgan BB. Workload, communication, and team structure in team performance. *Mil Psychol.* 1995;72(2):123-139.

17. Morley L, Cashell A. Collaboration in healthcare. *J Med Imag Radiat Sci.* 2017;48:207-216.

18. Tuckman BW. Developmental sequence in small groups. *Psychol Bull.* 1965;63:384-399.

19. Tuckman BW, Jensen MAC. Stages of small group development revisited. *Group Organ Stud.* 1977;2(4):419-427.

20. Sullivan TJ. *Collaboration: A Health Care Imperative.* New York, NY: McGraw-Hill; 1998.

21. Institute of Medicine Committee on Measuring the Impact of Interprofessional Education on Collaborative Practice and Patient Outcomes. *Measuring the Impact of Interprofessional Education on Collaboration Practice and Patient Outcomes.* Washington DC: National Academies Press; 2015.

22. Brandt B, Lutfiyya MN. Interprofessional practice, research and education. http://webfiles.anpd.org/InterprofessionalPracticeResearchEducation.mp4. Published 2015. Accessed November 18, 2018.

23. Hardin L, Kilian A, Spykerman K. Competing health care systems and complex patients: an interprofessional collaboration to improve outcomes and reduce health care costs. *J Interprof Educ Pract.* 2017;7:5-10.

24. Almkuist K. Pharmacist-nurse collaboration: decreasing 30-day readmissions for heart failure. *MEDSURG Nurs.* 2018;27(3):187-200.

25. Reeves S, Perrier L, Goldman J, Freeth D, Zwarenstein M. Interprofessional education: effects on professional practice and healthcare outcomes (update). *Cochrane Database Syst Rev.* 2013(3):CD002213.

26. Brashers V, Owen J, Haizlip J. Interprofessional education and practice guide no. 2: developing and implementing a center for interprofessional education. *J Interprof Care.* 2015;29(2):95-99.

27. Scoville R, Little K, Rakover J, Luther K, Mate K. *Sustaining Improvement. IHI White Paper.* Cambridge, MA: Institute for Healthcare Improvement; 2016.

28. National Conference of State Legislatures. The Medical Home Model of Care. www.ncsl.org/research/health/the-medical-home-model-of-care.aspx. Published 2012. Accessed November 14, 2018.

29. Emory News Center. Emory Saint Joseph's introduces new model of patient care. http://news.emory.edu/stories/2015/03/saint_josephs_SIBR/. Published 2015. Accessed November 18, 2018.

30. Cline E, Sweeny NL, Cooper PB. Medical home model: reducing cost, increasing care, and improving outcomes for uninsured, chronically ill patients. *Nurs Econ.* 2018;36(6):7-11, 28.

31. Ong I, Dino M, Calimag N, Hidalo F. Development and validation of interprofessional learning assessment tool for health professionals in continuing professional development (CPD). Jan 25, 2019;14(1). doi:10.1371/journal.pone.0211405. eCollection 2019.

32. American Institutes for Research. TeamSTEPPS Teamwork Perceptions Questionnaire (T-TPQ) Manual. 2010. Washington, DC: American Institutes for Research.

Chapter 7

1. Borkowski N. *Organizational Behavior in Health Care.* 3rd ed. Burlington, MA: Jones & Bartlett Learning; 2016.

2. Hicks JM. Leader communication styles and organizational health. *Health Care Manag.* 2011;30(1):86-91. doi:10.1097/HCM.0b013e3182078bf8

3. Soubhi H. Toward an experiential approach to interprofessional communication. *J Res Interprof Pract Educ.* 2017;7(1):1-3. https://ucark.idm.oclc.org/login?url=https://search.ebscohost.com/login.aspx?direct=true&db=a9h&AN=126590330&site=ehost-live&scope=site.

4. Askay D. Communication. In: Levi D, ed. *Group Dynamics for Teams.* 5th ed. Los Angeles, CA: Sage; 2016.

5. Hulit LM, Fahey KR, Howard MR. *Born to Talk: An Introduction to Speech and Language Development.* 6th ed. Boston, MA: Pearson Education; 2015.

6. Lake D, Baerg K, Paslawski T. *Teamwork, Leadership and Communication: Collaboration Basics for Health Professionals.* Edmonton, Alberta: Brush Education Inc; 2015.

7. Nelson DL, Quick JC. *Organizational Behavior: Foundations, Realities, and Challenges.* 4th ed. Mason, OH: South-Western College Pub; 2003.

8. Mehrabian A. *Silent Messages: Implicit Communication of Emotions and Attitudes.* 2nd ed. Belmont, CA; 1980.

9. Chandler D. *Semantics: The Basics.* 2nd ed. New York, NY: Routledge; 2007.

10. Duffy FD, Gordon GH, Whelan G, Cole-Kelly K, Frankel R. Assessing competence in communication and interpersonal skills: the Kalamazoo II report. *Acad Med.* 2004;79(6):495-507. https://ucark.idm.oclc.org/login?url=https://search.ebscohost.com/login.aspx?direct=true&db=cmedm&AN=15165967&site=ehost-live&scope=site.

11. Klinzing DR, Klinzing DG. *Communication for Allied Health Professionals.* Dubuque, IA: Wm C Brown; 1985.

12. Interprofessional Education Collaborative (IPEC) Expert Panel. *Core Competencies for Interprofessional Collaborative Practice: Report of an Expert Panel.* Washington, DC: IPEC; 2011.

13. Lustig MW, Koester J. *Intercultural Competence: Interpersonal Communication Across Cultures.* 6th ed. Boston, MA: Allyn and Bacon; 2006.

14. Kaderavek JN. *Language Disorders in Children: Fundamental Concepts of Assessment and Intervention.* Boston, MA: Allyn & Bacon; 2011.

15. Taylor O. Language and language differences. In: Anderson N, Shames G, eds. *Human Communication Disorders.* 3rd ed. Upper Saddle River, NJ: Merrill/Prentice Hall; 1990.

16. Tannen D. *You Just Don't Understand: Women and Men in Conversation.* New York, NY: William Morrow & Co; 1990.

17. Podesta JS. Gender games. *People.* 1994;42(15):71.

18. Burch V. Interprofessional education—is it "chakalaka" medicine? *Afr J Health Prof Educ.* 2014;6(1):2. doi:10.7196/AJHPE.424

19. McNair RP. The case for educating health care students in professionalism as the core content of interprofessional education. *Med Educ.* 2005;39(5):456-464. doi:10.1111/j.1365-2929.2005.02116.x.

20. Seery L. Top 10 essential skills for effective communication. Skillsology. https://skillsology.com/wc/top-10-essential-skills-for-effective-communication. Published 2016. Accessed September 19, 2019.

21. Johnson RH, Macpherson CF, Smith AW, Block RG, Keyton J. Facilitating teamwork in adolescent and young adult oncology. *J Oncol Pract.* 2016;12(11):1067-1074. doi:10.1200.JOP.2016.013870.

22. McNaughton D, Vostal BR. Using active listening to improve collaboration with parents: the LAFF don't CRY strategy. *Interv Sch Clin.* 2010;45(4):251-256. https://doi-org.ucark.idm.oclc.org/10.1177/1053451209353443

23. Lee SY, Dong L, Lim YH, Poh CL, Lim WS. SBAR: towards a common interprofessional team-based communication tool. *Med Educ.* 2016;50(11):1167-1168. https://doi-org.ucark.idm.oclc.org/10.1111/medu.13171

24. Hawkins P, Shohet R. *Supervision in the helping professions.* 3rd ed. Berkshire, UK: Open University Press; 2006.

25. Motley V, Reese MK, Campos P. Evaluating corrective feedback self-efficacy changes among counselor educators and site supervisors. *Couns Educ Superv.* 2014;53(1):34-46. https://doi-org.ucark.idm.oclc.org/10.1002/j.1556-6978.2014.00047.x

26. Rashotte J, Varpio L, Day K, et al. Mapping communication spaces: the development and use for analyzing the impact of EHRs on interprofessional collaborative practice. *Int J Med Inform.* 2016;93:2:2-13. doi:10.1016/j.ijmedinf.2016.05.003

27. Sheehan, D, Robertson, L, Ormond, T. Comparison of language used and patterns of communication in interprofessional and multidisciplinary teams. *J Interprof Care.* 2007;21(1):17-30.

Chapter 8

1. Centers for Medicare and Medicaid Services (CMS). Accountable care organizations. www.cms.gov/Medicare/Medicare-Fee-for-Service-Payment/ACO/. Updated May 3, 2018. Accessed November 11, 2018.

2. United Nations (UN). *Report of the World Commission on Environment and Development* (42/187). https://digitallibrary.un.org/record/153026. Published December 11, 1987. Accessed November 11, 2018.

3. Barbier EB. The concept of sustainable economic development. *Environ Conserv.* 1987;14(2):101-110. doi:10.1017/S0376892900011449

4. Fineberg HV. A successful and sustainable health system—how to get there from here. *N Engl J Med.* 2012;366:1020-1027. doi:10.1056/NEJMsa1114777

5. World Health Organization (WHO). *World Report on Knowledge for Better Health: Strengthening Health Systems.* www.who.int/rpc/meetings/en/world_report_on_knowledge_for_better_health2.pdf. Published 2004. Accessed November 11, 2018.

6. Balas EA, Boren SA. Managing clinical knowledge for health care improvement. *Yearb Med Inform.* 2000;(1):65-70.

7. Lawlis TR, Anson J, Greenfield D. Barriers and enablers that influence sustainable interprofessional education: a literature review. *J Interprof Care.* 2014;28(4):305-310.

8. National Academy of Medicine (NAM). Measuring the impact of interprofessional education on collaborative practice and patient outcomes. www.nap.edu/download/21726#. Published 2015. Accessed November 11, 2018.

9. Pullon S, Morgan S, Macdonald L, McKinlay E, Gray B. Observation of interprofessional collaboration in primary care practice: a multiple case study. *J Interprof Care.* 2016;30(6):787-794. doi:10.1080/13561820.2016.1220929

10. National Academy of Medicine (NAM). Press release: Institute of Medicine to become National Academy of Medicine. www.nationalacademies.org/hmd/Global/News%20Announcements/IOM-to-become-NAM-Press-Release.aspx. Published April 28, 2015. Accessed November 11, 2018.

11. National Academy of Medicine (NAM). Educating for the health team. https://nexusipe-resource-exchange.s3-us-west-2.amazonaws.com/Educating_for_the_Health_Team_IOM_1972.pdf. Published October 1972. Accessed November 11, 2018.

12. World Health Organization (WHO). Framework for Action on Interprofessional Education and Collaborative Practice. http://apps.who.int/iris/bitstream/handle/10665/70185/WHO_HRH_HPN_10.3_eng.pdf;jsessionid=67F6212E486D2BF3E03C796554F6267B?sequence=1. Published 2010. Accessed November 11, 2018.

13. Health Professions Accreditors Collaborative (HPAC). Home. http://healthprofessionsaccreditors.org/. Accessed November 11, 2018.

14. Health Professions Accreditors Collaborative (HPAC). Members. http://healthprofessionsaccreditors.org/members/. Accessed November 11, 2018.

15. National Academy of Medicine (NAM). *Health Professions Education: A Bridge to Quality.* www.nap.edu/download/10681. Published March 2003. Accessed November 11, 2018.

16. Rosalind Franklin University of Medicine and Science. College of Health Professions. www.rosalindfranklin.edu/academics/college-of-health-professions/degree-programs/interprofessional-healthcare-studies-phd/. Accessed November 11, 2018.

17. University of California San Francisco. Healthcare Administration and Interprofessional Leadership Program. https://healthleadership.ucsf.edu/. Accessed November 11, 2018.

18. Joint Accreditation for Interprofessional Continuing Education. About Joint Accreditation. www.jointaccreditation.org. Accessed November 11, 2018.

19. Joint Accreditation for Interprofessional Continuing Education. Accredited providers. www.jointaccreditation.org/accredited-providers. Accessed November 11, 2018.

20. Interprofessional Education Collaborative (IPEC). Resources. www.ipecollaborative.org/resources.html. Accessed November 12, 2018.

21. Josiah Macy Jr. Foundation. Publications: interprofessional education and teamwork. https://macyfoundation.org/assets/reports/publications/jmf_ipe_book_web.pdf. Accessed November 12, 2018.

22. National Academy of Medicine (NAM). Core principles and values of effective team-based health care. https://nam.edu/wp-content/uploads/2015/06/VSRT-Team-Based-Care-Principles-Values.pdf. Published October 2012. Accessed November 12, 2018.

23. National Academy of Medicine (NAM). Interprofessional education for collaboration: learning how to improve health from interprofessional models across the continuum of education to practice—workshop summary. www.nap.edu/download/13486#. Published 2013. Accessed November 12, 2018.

24. Robert Wood Johnson Foundation (RWJF). Lessons from the field: promising interprofessional collaboration practices. www.rwjf.org/en/library/research/2015/03/lessons-from-the-field.html. Published March 10, 2015. Accessed November 12, 2018.

25. World Health Organization (WHO). Interprofessional collaborative practice in primary health care: nursing and midwifery perspectives. www.who.int/hrh/resources/observer13/en/. Published September 2013. Accessed November 12, 2018.

26. World Health Organization (WHO). Interprofessional collaborative practice in primary health care: nursing and midwifery perspectives, six case studies. www.who.int/hrh/resources/IPE_SixCaseStudies.pdf. Published 2013. Accessed November 12, 2018.

27. Health Resources and Services Administration (HRSA). News and events: HRSA press releases. New coordinating center will promote interprofessional education and collaborative practice in health care. www.hrsa.gov/about/news/press-releases/2012-09-14-interprofessional.html. Published September 14, 2012. Accessed November 11, 2018.

28. Agency for Healthcare Research and Quality (AHRQ). About TeamSTEPPS. www.ahrq.gov/teamstepps/about-teamstepps/index.html. Published August 2015. Updated April 2017. Accessed November 11, 2018.

29. Farnsworth TJ, Peterson T, Neill K, Neill M, Sikel JA, Lawson J. Understanding the structural, human resource, political, and symbolic dimensions of implementing and sustaining interprofessional education. *J Allied Health*. 2015;44(3):152-157.

30. Hammick M, Freeth D, Koppel I, Reeves, Barr H. A best evidence systematic review of interprofessional education: BEME Guide no. 9. *Med Teach*. 2007;29(8):735-751. doi:10.1080/01421590701682576.

31. Josiah Macy Jr. Foundation. Transforming patient care: aligning interprofessional education with clinical practice redesign. ww.w.macyfoundation.org/docs/macy_pubs/JMF_TransformingPatientCare_Jan2013Conference_fin_Web.pdf#page=115. Published January 2013. Accessed November 11, 2018.

32. D'Amour D, Oandasan I. Interprofessionality as the field of interprofessional practice and interprofessional education: an emerging concept. *J Inteprof Care*. 2005;19(S1):8-20.

33. Grymonpre RE, Ateah CA, Dean HJ, et al. Sustainable implementation of interprofessional education using an adoption model framework. *Can J Higher Ed*. 2016;46(4):76-93.

34. Hall LW, Zierler BK. Interprofessional education and practice guide no.1: developing faculty to effectively facilitate interprofessional education. *J Inteprof Care*. 2015;29(1):3-7. doi:10.3109/13561820.2014.937483

35. Olson RE, Klupp N, Astell-Burt T. Reimagining health professional socialisation: an interactionist study of interprofessional education. *Health Sociol Rev*. 2016;25(1):92-107.

36. Holland D, Lachicotte W, Skinner D, Cain C. *Identity and Agency in Cultural Worlds*. Cambridge, MA: Harvard University Press; 1998.

37. Carney PA, Bearden DT, Osborne ML, et al. Economic models for sustainable interprofessional education. *J Inteprof Care*. 2018;32(6):745-751. doi:10.1080/13561820.2018.1509846.

38. Health Professions Accreditors Collaborative (HPAC). *Guidance on Developing Quality Interprofessional Education for the Health Professions*. https://nexusipe-summit.s3.us-west-2.amazonaws.com/2019/2019-01/HPAC-National-Center-GuidanceWeb-1.pdf. Accessed June 26, 2019.

39. National Collaborative for Improving the Clinical Learning Environment. *Achieving the Optimal Interprofessional Clinical Learning Environment*. https://storage.googleapis.com/wzukusers/user-27661272/documents/5c51b3628dae7ExACzM9/1071%20NCICLE%20IP-CLE%20SymPro%20Booklet-DIGITAL%20FINAL.pdf. Accessed September 5, 2019.

40. Reinders J, Pesut D, Brocklehurst P, Paans W, van der Schans C. Meta-model of interprofessional development. www.youtube.com/watch?v=uj9Csu1jvlY. Accessed September 26, 2019.

41. Salas E, Lazzara E, Benishek L, King H. On being a team player: Evidence-based heuristic for teamwork in interprofessional education. *Med Sci Educ*. 2013;23(3S):524-531.

42. Salas E. Saving lives: The science of teamwork and what matters in practice. Presentation at Louisiana State University Health-New Orleans.

43. The Global Network for Interprofessional Education and Collaborative Practice Research. *Guidance on Global Interprofessional Education and Collaborative Practice Research: Discussion Paper*. https://research.interprofessional.global/wp-content/uploads/2019/10/Guidance-on-Global-Interprofessional-Education-and-Collaborative-Practice-Research_Discussion-Paper_FINAL-WEB.pdf. Accessed November 3, 2019.

44. National Academy of Medicine (NAM). *Strengthening the Connection between Health Professions Education and Practice: Proceedings of a Joint Workshop*. http://nationalacademies.org/hmd/Reports/2019/strengthening-connection-between-health-professions-education-practice-proceedings.aspx. Accessed November 5, 2019.

45. Interprofessional Education–The Genesis of Global Movement. https://www.caipe.org/resources/publications/caipe-publications/caipe-2015-interprofessional-education-genesis-global-movement-barr-h. Accessed November 10, 2019.

46. Interprofessional Education Guidelines. https://www.caipe.org/resources/publications/caipe-publications/caipe-2017-interprofessional-education-guidelines-barr-h-ford-j-gray-r-helme-m-hutchings-m-low-h-machin-reeves-s. Accessed November 10, 2019.

47. CAIPE Fellows Statement on Integrative Care. https://www.caipe.org/resources/publications/caipe-publications/lindqvist-s-anderson-e-diack-l-reeves-s-2017-caipe-fellows-statement-integrative-care. Accessed November 10, 2019.

48. Khalili H. Towards the Development of Dual Identity through Interprofessional Socialization: A Critical Reflective Analysis. Accepted for Oral Presentation, Collaborating Across Borders VII (CAB VII) Conference, Indianapolis, Indiana. October 20-22, 2019.

49. Khalili H. Interprofessional socialization and dual identity development amongst cross-disciplinary students. Dissertation, University of Western Ontario, London, Canada. 2013.

50. Khalili H, Orchard C, Laschinger HK, Farah R. An interprofessional socialization framework for developing an interprofessional identity among health professions students. *J Interprof Care.* 2013;27(6), 448-453.

51. Pettigrew TF. Intergroup contact theory. *Annual Review of Psychology.* 1998;49(1), 65–85.

52. Canadian Interprofessional Health Collaborative (CIHC) Competencies Working Group. *A National Interprofessional Competency Framework.* Vancouver, BC: Canadian Interprofessional Health Collaborative. http://www.cihc.ca/files/CIHC_IPCompetencies_Feb1210.pdf.

53. Interprofessional Education Collaborative. *Core competencies for interprofessional collaborative practice: 2016 update.* Washington, DC: Author. https://ipecollaborative.org/uploads/IPEC-2016-Updated-Core-Competencies-Report__final_release_.PDF.

Index

Note: The italicized *f* and *t* following page numbers refer to figures and tables, respectively.

About the Editors

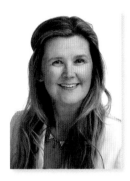

Jordan Hamson-Utley, PhD, LAT, ATC, is the director of the postprofessional master of health science program and an associate professor at the University of St. Augustine for Health Sciences, where she presides as chairperson of the interprofessional education task force. Utley has practiced as a certified athletic trainer for 25 years across various settings and has 20 years of experience in health sciences education and academic leadership. She serves as a committee member of the National Athletic Trainers' Association Post-Professional Education Committee (PPEC) and on the program planning committee for the American Interprofessional Health Collaborative (AIHC).

Utley was awarded Apple's Distinguished Educator award in 2012 for innovative use of technology in health care education. She received the Excellence in Publishing Award from the University of Phoenix in 2014. In 2016, Utley was recognized for her collaboration and leadership at the University of St. Augustine when she accepted the Stanley Paris Award, the highest honor awarded by the board to university faculty members. In 2019, the National Athletic Trainers' Association awarded her the International Speaker Grant to present on the impact of interprofessional education in health care.

Utley is a coauthor of the book *Psychosocial Strategies for Athletic Training* and continues to promote the evolving role of the athletic trainer on the health care team. Photo © University of St. Augustine for Health Sciences.

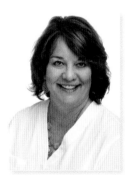

Cynthia Kay Mathena, PhD, OTR/L, is the dean of the College of Health Sciences at the University of St. Augustine for Health Sciences. Her responsibilities include oversight of programs with a focus on interprofessional education and innovative online delivery.

Mathena has over 30 years of experience as an occupational therapist and 25 years of higher education experience. She is active in state, local, and national professional organizations and serves on accreditation site visit teams as a chair. She has recently published on topics that include service learning and online education and has presented nationally on simulation and on approaches to interprofessional education. In her free time, she enjoys outdoor activities, fitness, and nutrition. Photo © University of St. Augustine for Health Sciences and Cynthia K. Mathena.

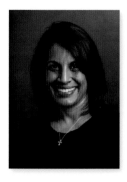

Tina Patel Gunaldo, PHD, DPT, MHS, is the director for the Center for Interprofessional Education and Collaborative Practice at Louisiana State University Health–New Orleans. In addition to presentations and publications, Dr. Gunaldo's professional contributions include serving on the American Interprofessional Health Collaborative's Scholarship Committee; on the Louisiana Immunization Workgroup, supporting a collaborative approach to increasing immunization rates; and on the American Physical Therapy Association's Finance Committee. She contributes to the development of the Scholars Program for the Louisiana Area Health Education Center (AHEC). She is also the coeditor of the *Health, Interprofessional Practice and Education* journal. Photo © Tina Patel Gunaldo.

Contributors

Anthony Breitbach, PhD, ATC, FASAHP
Saint Louis University

Robin Dennison, DNP, APRN, CCNS, NEA-BC
University of St. Augustine for Health Sciences

Joy Doll, OTD, OTR/L
Creighton University

Kathrin Eliot, PhD, RD, FAND
University of Oklahoma Health Sciences Center

Amy Herrington, DNP, RN, CEN, CNE
University of St. Augustine for Health Sciences

K. Michelle Knewstep-Watkins, OTD, OTR/L
Mary Baldwin University and University of Virginia Health System

Dee M. Lance, PhD, CCC-SLP/L
University of Central Arkansas

Melanie Logue, PhD, DNP, APRN, CFNP, FAANP
University of St. Augustine for Health Sciences

C. Michelle Longley, MSN, RN, NP-C
University of Virginia Health System

Kim C. McCullough, PhD, CCC-SLP/L
Appalachian State University

Meghan M. Scanlon, BSIE
Six Sigma Black Belt and Value Capture

Judi Schack-Dugré, PT, DPT, MBA, EdD
University of Florida

Pamela Waynick-Rogers, DNP, APRN-BC
Vanderbilt University

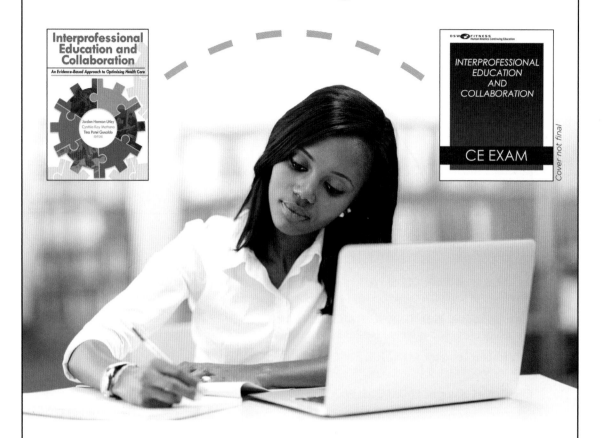
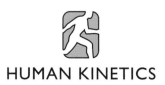